Difficult Consultations with Adolescents

Chris Donovan
and
Heather C Suckling
with
Zoe Walker
Janet Bell
Tami Kramer
Sheila R Cross

Radcliffe Medical Press
Oxford • San Francisco

Radcliffe Medical Press Ltd
18 Marcham Road
Abingdon
Oxon OX14 1AA
United Kingdom

www.radcliffe-oxford.com
The Radcliffe Medical Press electronic catalogue and online ordering facility.
Direct sales to anywhere in the world.

_____

British Library Cataloguing in Publication Data

A catalogue record for this book is available from the British Library.

ISBN 1 85775 882X

Typeset by Action Publishing Technology Ltd, Gloucester
Printed and bound by TJ International Ltd, Padstow, Cornwall

Contents

Foreword

It is a great pleasure for me to be able to write a foreword to this unusual and important book. Through my involvement with the Royal College of General Practitioners Adolescent Task Group, I have been aware of and impressed by the project on difficult consultations. From the outset I had no doubt that this was an area of work which urgently needed attention, yet rarely received it. Research tells us that in their consultations GPs find teenage patients less easy to deal with than any other age group. How much more difficult must it be when the young person is troubled, embarrassed, awkward, angry, resentful or just simply uncommunicative? This book, which is a report based on the project set up and inspired by Dr Chris Donovan, will prove an invaluable resource for all those working in the field of primary healthcare and family medicine.

The book represents a plea for a better understanding of the special needs of young people in their dealings with doctors and other healthcare professionals. Through the case histories the reader will be introduced to adolescents who are depressed, to those who have been failed by the system, to those who cannot communicate their needs, and to those for whom issues of confidentiality have become critical. We can reasonably hope that, by reading this book, adults working with young people can come to a greater awareness of the circumstances of the adolescent patient. We can also hope that, through this increased awareness, changes in practice can be made so that teenagers are able to receive healthcare which is appropriate to their needs. However, there is more in this book than simply a call for a better understanding of young people. The reader will also learn about the professional's perspective, and through this they can recognise that working with adolescents is not always easy. The professional also needs assistance to enable them to do a good job with young people. More training in this field should be a priority, and the publication of this material should offer ammunition for those arguing this particular case.

I have no doubt that this book will prove an exceptional resource over the coming years. It should be required reading for those in training, and should provide invaluable material for those designing training courses for health professionals working with young people. I am delighted to have been associated with this project, and to have shared in some small measure with Chris Donovan and his colleagues their passionate commitment to better healthcare for all young people in our society. I wish the book every success.

John Coleman
December 2003

Foreword

'Confidentiality at the doctors means he can't tell anyone what you say, your mum, your family, no one, but you think he won't tell anyone, well you hope he won't!'

'What you say to the doctor is supposed to be confidential, but does this apply especially if they know your family, you don't know what they'd let slip!'

'The doctor said I was in a dangerous state – I don't know what he means'

'My sister's very depressed, the doctor won't listen to me. He's given her sleeping pills, how stupid can you get?'

'I can't tell my GP – he plays golf with my Dad'

These are all quotes from young people about their doctors. It is worth noting that, contrary to popular belief, young people on average visit their GPs three or four times a year. These visits provide opportunities for a sensitive approach, and permit a range of issues to be explored, revealing something that may not be immediately apparent. There may also be concerns that are too embarrassing for young people to 'bring up' spontaneously by themselves – such as sex, relationships, depression or feelings of inadequacy.

This is not to say that many, even most, consultations with young people will be easy and uncomplicated. But there will also be occasions when the consultation may be difficult and challenging both for young people and health professionals alike.

Not surprisingly there are rarely perfect answers as to how these problems should be dealt with. Rather, there are better or worse ways of approaching them. However, it is important not to assume that all teenagers have complex unsolved needs. Most young people go through their teenage years unscathed and emerge as adults, having experimented with sex, drugs and tobacco, and equipped to deal with the vicissitudes of adult life, still talking to their parents and making appropriate use of the available social and medical services.

This book offers ideas, insights and ways in which the different issues affecting young people can be discussed and dealt with. From the silent to the aggressive; from the embarrassed to the anxious; from the simple to the difficult; from the confused to the depressed, there are chapters here which look at real-life consultations from the viewpoints of doctors, nurses, parents and teenagers. It is a book for anyone who cares for and is interested in teenagers, and for those who are also dedicated to delivering better services.

Although adolescents have managed to survive (as adults we bear testament to this), 'survival' alone is now not enough. We want troubled teenagers to be welcomed when they need help, to feel that general practice is approachable, and that their problems will not only be heard, but taken seriously and dealt with in the most effective way possible.

This book will help us to do all these things.

Ann McPherson
December 2003

About the authors

Chris Donovan MA (Oxon) FRCGP worked as a general practitioner in North London for over 30 years. He was a trainer, course organiser and chair of the part time senior GP lecturers at The Royal Free Medical School. Twelve years ago he founded and chaired the RCGP Task Group. After leaving the practice he worked as a part time consultant at Great Ormond Street Hospital in their long-term follow-up cancer clinic and was medical adviser at Coram Family. He is currently chair of Brent Centre for Young People, is on the council of Young Minds and the board of The Trust for the Study of Adolescence (TSA) and is honorary senior lecturer in the Centre for Community Child Health at The Royal Free.

Heather C Suckling FRCGP worked as a general practitioner in Islington, London for more than 34 years. She was course organiser for the Homerton and St Bartholomew's General Practice Vocational Training Scheme for 15 years and was chairperson of the National Association of Course Organisers from 1991–1994. She has been a Balint group leader for 23 years and was president of the Balint Society from 1999–2003. She is now the general secretary of the International Balint Federation. She is leading a Balint group for the first clinical year medical students at The Royal Free and University College Medical School where she also teaches professional development to first and second year medical students.

Zoe Walker was the principal researcher at the Department of Primary Care, University of Hertfordshire, under Professor Joy Townsend. Zoe chaired the steering committee of the Adolescent Consultations Evaluated (ACE) project, where she met Dr Chris Donovan and Janet Bell. She later became a significant contributor to the project described in this book. Zoe was a member of the editorial team for the project until her untimely death at the age of 31 years. Just a few days before she died, she was awarded her PhD from the University of Hertfordshire as a result of her work on adolescent consultations. Zoe is survived by her husband Dr Robin Walker and their son Alex, born in September 1999.

Janet Bell RGB BSc (Hons) GCE is a nurse practitioner working in general practice in Hertfordshire. She is also employed by the local PCT as a primary care tutor supporting practice nurses in their continuing professional development. In 1994 she started inviting teenagers to attend the surgery for health promotion consultations. As a result of this work, she worked closely with Zoe Walker on the ACE project, being a member of the steering group and interviewing the teenagers in the intervention consultation. Janet is currently involved with another research project involving teenagers, looking at an intervention to encourage physical activity.

Tami Kramer works as a consultant child and adolescent psychiatrist for Central and North West London Mental Health Trust and as a senior clinical research fellow at Imperial College, London. She has a special interest in adolescent mental health. Her current research interests include the development of evidence-based services for adolescents, adolescent depression and the role of primary care, the link between physical and emotional symptoms, refugee mental health and the use of outcome measures.

Sheila R Cross was consultant paediatrician in a North London Hospital. Since retiring ten years ago she has worked as a volunteer at ChildLine. She works regularly as a telephone counsellor and as a trainer of new volunteers. She has researched and written three reports for ChildLine: *I Know You're Not a Doctor But ...* describes calls from young people about their own health and the health of people close to them. *Can You Get it From Toothpaste?* tells of the anxieties experienced by children from a wide age range about HIV and AIDS. *I Can't Stop Feeling Sad* tells the stories of children trying to cope with grief after a bereavement.

John Coleman is a chartered psychologist and a Fellow of the British Psychological Society. He has been the director of the Trust for the Study of Adolescence since 1989. He has written widely about adolescence, one of his most well-known books being *The Nature of Adolescence*, the third edition of which was co-authored with Leo Hendry and published by Routledge in 1999. He was the editor of the *Journal of Adolescence* from 1984 to 2000, and he has carried out research on young people and mental health.

Ann McPherson has worked as a general practitioner in Oxford since 1979. She is a fellow of Green College, Oxford and a lecturer in the Department of General Practice at Oxford University where she researches into adolescent health and patients' experiences of illness (www.dipex.org). With Aidan Macfarlane, she had authored several books for teenagers including *The Teenage Health Freak* series and runs a teenage web site www.teenagehealth-freak.org which gives health information to young people in an innovative way including a virtual on-line surgery. With Chris Donovan, she has co-written a training manual and confidentiality toolkit to improve teenage health in general practice. She is chairperson of the Adolescent Task Force of the Royal College of General Practitioners.

Dedication

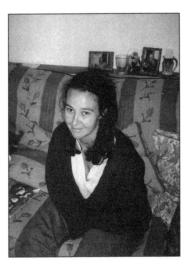

Zoe Alice Katherine Walker
15 February 1970 – 10 September 2001

This book is dedicated to the memory of our colleague
Dr Zoe Walker.

Acknowledgements

This book was inspired by a project undertaken by the RCGP Adolescent Task Group
   We would like to thank the following:

- all those who participated in the discussion groups for this project and who offered their expertise and gave so freely of their time. Without their work, this book could not have been written. We feel that their names should not be disclosed but we would like to offer them our particular thanks
- the members of the RCGP Task Group, especially Dr Dick Churchill, Dr Marion Davies and Dr Aidan Macfarlane, who commented on the first draft of this book. We especially appreciated the detailed comments made by Dr Lionel Jacobson
- the Omega Foundation, which provided a grant to support the work of writing up the results
- the Royal College of General Practitioners, for providing a meeting room and refreshments
- Mrs Sheila Austin for transcribing the tapes.

The Omega Foundation

25 Middleway
London NW11 6SH

The Omega Foundation was established in 1987 by Dr Susan Bach. It provides grants to assist research into methods of alleviating the suffering of seriously ill patients who are affected by physical or psychiatric conditions. One of its aims is to support projects designed to improve the skills of health professionals. The Foundation is concerned with the needs of both children and adults.

The RCGP Adolescent Task Group

The Adolescent Task Group (formerly the Adolescent Working Party) is a multidisciplinary group that was formed in the early 1990s to promote the needs of young people in primary care.

Its aim is to promote improved quality of general-practice-based primary care medical services in relation to meeting the health needs of young people aged 11–19 years during the transition to adulthood.

Task Group members are all involved in education, research or service provision related to young people. For further details, visit www.rcgp.org.uk. The composition of the Task Group at the time the project was started (left hand column) and at the time of publication (right hand column), was as follows.

Chair

Dr Chris Donovan

Members

Dr Richard Burack
Professor Ruth Chambers
Dr Dick Churchill
Dr John Coleman
Dr Marian Davis
Professor Elena Garralda
Dr Lionel Jacobson
Dr Aidan Macfarlane
Dr Ann McPherson
Judy McRae
Sara Richards
Dr Hilary Smith

Chair

Dr Ann McPherson

Members

Dr Richard Burack
Professor Ruth Chambers
Dr Dick Churchill
Dr John Coleman
Dr Marian Davis
Dr Chris Donovan
Professor Elena Garralda
Mary Gyte
Dr Lionel Jacobson
Elaine Lunts
Dr Aidan Macfarlane
Judy McRae
Kathy Phipps
Sara Richards
Dr Hilary Smith
Helen Stokes-Lampard

Introduction

World Health Organization definitions

Children   0–18 years of age
Adolescents   10–19 years of age
Young people   10–25 years of age
Youth   15–25 years of age

Source: Coleman and Schofield.[1]

Statistics

- Children and adolescents (0- to 19-year-olds) represent a quarter of the UK population, with a total of 7.5 million adolescents.
- There were 3.9 million adolescents aged 10–14 years in the UK in 2001.
- There were 3.6 million adolescents aged 15–19 years in the UK in 2001.
- Adolescents visit a GP two or three times a year on average. Over 80% of all adolescents see their GP at least once a year.

The health of adolescents and finding better ways to meet their physical and mental health needs are matters of national and international concern.

Key facts about adolescent health

- There has been a recent reduction in the rate of pregnancy among those under 18 years of age in the UK, however the UK rate is still the highest in Europe. In 2000, the rate for the 15–17 years age group was 16.6 per 1000 females.
- The incidence of sexually transmitted infections among young people has risen markedly in the UK during the last decade. The number of new diagnoses of chlamydia and gonorrhoea among 16- to 19-year-olds more than doubled between 1996 and 2001.
- Mortality did not fall among 15- to19-year-olds or 20- to 24-year-olds in the UK during the last decade, although it did in all other age groups.
- Among 5- to 15-year-olds, 20% of males and 15% of females rate themselves as having a long-standing illness. Around 15% of adolescents suffer from some form of psychiatric problem.
- Among 15- to 24-year-old males in the UK, approximately 550 commit suicide each year. The rates are higher in Scotland and Northern Ireland than in England

and Wales. It is estimated that around 20 000 young people in this age group are admitted to hospital each year as a result of self-harm.
- Alcohol consumption has risen among young people over the last decade in the UK. The amount consumed per week has doubled among the 11–15 years age group, and has increased by 80% among the 15–19 years age group.

There have always been strong humanitarian reasons for adults to support adolescents through their teenage years, in order to increase the chances of them climbing the ladder of emotional and educational development and reaching their potential as adults.

Now that the UK has an ageing population (with a higher percentage of over-65s than under-16s), there are also strong economic reasons for adults to provide teenage-friendly services for young people in trouble, in the hope that these services will help them to surmount their difficulties and so develop into responsible parents, concerned citizens and adult wealth creators.

These are some of the reasons why there is concern about improving the medical services that are available to this age group. Much of this concern is focused on the structure and outcome of these services.

What receives less attention, but is of equal importance, is the 'process' experienced by adolescents when they seek support for a personal problem, especially if they are unable or reluctant to share that problem with their families. In primary care, this process includes the way in which they acquire information about services, how easily they can access those services, how teenage-friendly the services are, and to what degree young people can trust those running the services to maintain confidentiality. All of these issues are gradually being addressed in many practices, but of equal importance is the way in which the consultation is conducted. This is the area that will be considered in this book.

The figures in the *Key facts* box on page xii suggest that many adolescent problems are not being dealt with adequately by our medical services. These problems are often those that are personally embarrassing to the patient, and which take time and sensitivity on the part of the health professional to unravel and sort out. Some research suggests that GPs do not always provide this extra time. In one study, consultations with adolescents were found to be two minutes shorter than those provided for adults,[2] possibly indicating that GPs do not explore many issues in great detail.[3] In a more recent study, over 20% of a sample of teenagers from the South Wales valleys commented that they do not have enough time in their consultations with GPs, and this correlates significantly with their overall measure of satisfaction with the consultation.[4]

In 1998, the Royal College of General Practitioners (RCGP) Adolescent Task Group organised a conference in London to look at adolescent consultations in primary care. Over 90 people attended, including GPs, practice nurses and other health professionals. Many participants felt that their adolescent contacts often proved difficult. Suggested explanations as to why this was the case included the following.

- A large number of adolescents have no experience of consulting on their own before going with an embarrassing personal problem to a GP or practice nurse whom they may only know as a friend of their family.
- Some adolescent problems include issues that the GP is not keen to hear about, either because they do not have the training necessary to deal with the problem, or because they

do not have the facilities to refer the patient on to secondary care. It is also possible that the problem may reactivate an unresolved problem in the professional's own life.

- Risk taking by patients in this age group with drugs, drink, sex and self-harm can irritate professionals, who feel that their efforts to care for their young patients are being unreasonably undermined by the patients themselves.

The conference agreed that these explanations were purely speculative. What was required was a detailed look at actual consultations which were thought to be difficult. It was hoped that if such research could be organised, it would reveal issues which would help GPs to conduct future consultations with this age group more successfully.

The Difficult Consultations with Adolescents project was therefore organised. This book has been inspired by the project, which is described in detail in Parts 1 and 2. We have maintained confidentiality by changing the names of patients and withholding the names of the professionals who participated.

The book is divided into six parts.

- Part 1 describes the project.
- Part 2 summarises the consultations that were discussed.
- Part 3 considers some of the factors that can make adolescent consultations difficult.
- Part 4 provides personal perspectives on consulting with adolescents from a GP, a practice nurse, a child and adolescent psychiatrist, and a paediatrician who has worked with ChildLine.
- Part 5 presents the conclusions.
- Part 6 provides suggestions for further reading.

The aim of the authors in producing this book is *not* to tell professionals how to conduct their consultations, but rather to stimulate discussion and thinking about the methods by which we might all improve our consulting skills with young people and reduce some of the difficult feelings that can arise from these contacts.

References

1 Coleman J and Schofield J (2003) *Key Data on Adolescence*. Trust for the Study of Adolescence, Brighton.
2 Jacobson LD and Owen P (1994) A study of teenage care in one general practice. *Br J Gen Pract.* **43**: 349.
3 Jacobson L, Wilkinson C and Owen P (1994) Is the potential of teenage consultations being missed? A study of consultation times in primary care. *Fam Pract.* **11**: 296–9.
4 Jacobson L, Richardson G, Parry-Langdon N *et al.* (2001) How do teenagers and primary healthcare providers view each other? An overview of key themes. *Br J Gen Pract.* **51**: 811–16.

Part 1

About the Difficult Consultations with Adolescents project

Chapter 1

Aims and methods of the project

Aims of the project

The primary aim of the project was to study some actual difficult consultations with adolescents, and the emotions engendered in the GP or practice nurse, in order to draw out themes that would shed light on the reasons why professionals label these consultations as 'difficult'. Our definition of a 'difficult consultation' was a consultation that the professional presenting remembered as being difficult for them.

(In this chapter we provide details of the research project so that readers who are interested in evidence can understand the context in which we heard the details of the consultations. For those who are concerned only with the consultations themselves, we recommend that you turn to Part 2, page 11.)

Choice of research method

It was clear that a qualitative rather than quantitative research method would be most appropriate for this project. This decision was supported by various authorities. For example, Pope and Mays have stated that qualitative research is an essential prerequisite of good quantitative research, particularly in areas where there has been little previous investigation.[1] Strong emphasises the value of qualitative methods in developing concepts to aid understanding of complex behaviours, attitudes and interactions.[2]

Which qualitative research method to use?

It was decided that group discussion would be used as the basis of the work. As the focus was to be on the interaction between the adolescent and the health professional and the emotions engendered, a Balint group was chosen. Hull refers to the use of a Balint group 'in capturing and amplifying the observation of the doctor/patient interaction revealed to the group.'[3] Harris described the Balint group as 'the only true ethnographic research that General Practice has evolved.'[4]

What is a Balint group?

A traditional Balint group consists of between six and ten GPs with one or two leaders. Originally the leaders were psychoanalysts, but now they are usually GPs. A recent development has been the introduction of multidisciplinary groups, which are becoming increasingly popular. The group meets regularly for one or two hours, usually weekly, for a period of one or more years. The membership is constant. Balint considered this to be essential in order to ensure that the group was 'safe' and the participants could build trust in each other. Confidentiality is implicit in any Balint group. (During our group sessions confidentiality was agreed, and in the reporting of cases all names have been changed to ensure anonymity of the patients and doctors involved.)

The leader opens the proceedings by asking 'Who has a case?', and one of the members then volunteers a presentation. This is not a traditional case presentation but the story of an encounter with a patient who for some reason continues to occupy the presenter's mind. No notes are used because, as in psychoanalysis, it is what is remembered (and forgotten) that is significant. After the initial presentation the group discusses the case, working together to try to understand the problem. The emphasis is on the relationship between the doctor and the patient, noting the emotions aroused and speculating about the possible reasons for these emotions. The aim is not to intrude on the doctor's inner world, but to recognise that the emotions engendered in the doctor and in the group may reflect the emotions in the patient, and to use these findings to aid diagnosis of the problem.

Balint, the doctor who developed the concept of Balint groups, concentrated on diagnosis rather than advice:

> 'Advice' is usually a well-intentioned shot in the dark, is nearly always futile and applies even more strongly to 'reassurance'. We have found it more profitable for both doctors and patients to diagnose the problem; more often than not, when that is done, there will be no need for either advice or reassurance. The real problem is likely to be unpleasant or even painful, but it will be real and with hard work it is probable that something real can be done about it.[5]

It can be difficult for a Balint group leader to avoid 'teaching' and to prevent the giving of 'advice' and 'reassurance', which come easily to health professionals as they form part of their traditional roles, but these may hamper a deeper exploration of the problem.

For details of the history of Balint groups, *see* Appendix 2.

Method

Participants

The Balint group for this project was multidisciplinary and consisted of the following:

- nine GPs
- one child/adolescent psychiatrist
- one healthcare researcher
- one health visitor
- one health promotion nurse.

One of the GPs (Dr Chris Donovan, the project director) had considerable experience of Balint work, and another (Dr Heather Suckling) was an accredited Balint leader, so these individuals were identified as the leaders of the group.

Because of the time and place of meetings, many of the original volunteers could not attend, and some new GPs were recruited.

Meetings

There were significant differences between the project group and a traditional Balint group. Only six meetings were held, and the group membership was not constant. The number attending each meeting ranged from six to nine. Five of the members, including the two leaders, attended all of the meetings. The meetings took place in 1998–99.

Refreshments were provided, as many of the participants came straight from their evening surgeries to the meetings.

Group rules

At the first meeting the ground rules were agreed, the need for confidentiality was emphasised, and the group's aims and objectives were confirmed (*see below*).

The leaders would like to comment that, despite the lack of constant membership of the group, a safe and trusting environment was established without difficulty from the beginning. This was a tribute to the commitment, experience and integrity of the group members.

Aim and objectives of the group

Aim
To improve communication between the doctor or healthcare worker and the adolescent by studying the interactions between them.

Objectives
- To look at actual consultations with particular reference to the doctor–patient or health worker–client relationship.
- To identify common themes or difficulties in the consultation.
- To identify feelings engendered by the consultation both in the doctor or healthcare worker and in the group.
- To draw together general themes which could be of help when conducting future consultations.

Presentations

The group members were asked to present only adolescent consultations which had proved difficult for them. After the presentation and a period of open group discussion, the group was asked to identify the following:

- feelings engendered in the presenter
- feelings engendered in the group

- themes and difficulties in this consultation
- themes that are common in consultations with adolescents.

This proved more complicated in practice than we had envisaged. To give the reader a feel for the process, we shall illustrate it by presenting the first case in Chapter 2.

In this study we chose to use a Balint group because of its ability to highlight the emotional aspects of the consultations, but we are aware of its limitations. In such groups, conclusions may only be drawn and interpretations made from the material that the presenter remembers and chooses to report, and from the subsequent speculations from members of the group. The readers, like the group members, will find that they are left with many unanswered questions. This reflects what will inevitably happen in their own consultations. This book is therefore not a 'how to do it' manual. However, if it opens the minds of its readers to new concerns and makes them question their consultation methods with young people, it will have achieved its aim.

We shall next present the first case that was discussed, in order to give the reader a feel for the process and an indication of how the various issues relating to adolescent consultations arose within the group.

References

1 Pope C and Mays N (1995) Researching the parts that other methods cannot reach: qualitative methods in health and health services research. *BMJ.* **311**: 42–5.
2 Strong P (1979) *The Ceremonial Order of the Clinic.* Routledge, London.
3 Hull S (1996) The method of Balint work and its contribution to research in general practice. *Fam Pract.* **13** (**Supplement 1**): 510–12.
4 Harris C (1989) Seeing sunflowers: the William Pickles lecture. *J R Coll Gen Pract.* **39**: 313–19.
5 Balint M (1957) *The Doctor, his Patient and the Illness.* Pitman Medical Press, London.

Chapter 2

Case A: 'Anne' – the adolescent who will not speak

Presenter:	GP: female, white, British.
Patient:	Anne (Case A): 13 years old, female, white, British.
Settings:	Five consultations in the practice.
	Visit to a child psychiatrist.
	Observed at home by the district nurse.
	These contacts took place over a period of several months.

What happened

- *Contact 1: Anne's mother phones the practice nurse during a teen clinic.*
  Anne's mother phoned to say that Anne was in tears, huddled in a chair and would not say what the problem was. The practice nurse suggested that Anne and her mother visit the surgery.
- *Contact 2: Anne visits the practice nurse at the teen clinic with her mother.*
  Anne remained in tears during the consultation and 'didn't really have a great deal to say'. The nurse suggested that when Anne went home she should try to tell her mother or sister what the problem was.
- *Contact 3: Anne visits the locum GP with her mother.*
  This was a long consultation. Anne was 'more communicative on this occasion'. She had refused to attend school for six weeks. There had been some bullying at school, and she had started her periods the preceding autumn. This was a traumatic time for her.
- *Contact 4: Anne visits the presenting GP with her mother and father. She is seen alone for part of the consultation.*
  Anne was anxious, short of breath and tearful. There was no eye contact. Anne sat half-facing her mother with her long hair hanging over her face, and she did not speak. Her mother did all of the talking. Anne's mother has myalgic encephalomyelitis (ME) and her father has multiple sclerosis (MS) which had been diagnosed two years previously. Anne has an older sister, aged 19 years, who lives locally.
  The GP saw Anne alone for a short time 'but she didn't say anything very much', so the GP continued to see her with her parents. Anne did not want her parents to leave, and was more tearful if they did so. The GP diagnosed that Anne was depressed and that 'something serious was going on'. Her response to a question about suicidal thoughts was a shrug.

The doctor decided that the nurse should visit Anne at home. She also referred her to a child psychiatrist and prescribed her antidepressants.

- *Contact 5: the district nurse observes Anne at home when she visits the family.*
  The nurse noted that Anne's father was in his wheelchair and had positioned himself where everyone had to walk past him.
- *Contact 6: Anne is taken to see a child psychiatrist by her parents (several times).*
  Anne did not want to go but eventually acquiesced. She did not communicate with the psychiatrist. He thought she might be suffering from ME, and referred her to a paediatrician.
- *Contact 7: Anne visits the presenting GP.*
  She seemed to be improving, and there was a 'hint of a smile'.
- *Contact 8: Anne visits the presenting GP with her mother and sister.*
  Anne's sister had now moved back into the family house. The presenting problem this time was Anne's periods, and it was thought that she wanted to go on the pill. Anne complained of tiredness and shortness of breath. She said she wanted to go to school but 'just can't do it'. As the psychiatrist had said he thought she might have ME, the GP took a blood test, although she was sure that it would be normal.

Doctor's feelings

- 'It is very difficult to communicate with someone if they won't speak to you.'
- 'Frustration is the biggest thing that I felt.'
- 'I arranged several things and gave her medication. I did very "doctory" things. I did things, which is what doctors do – they do things.'
- 'It was all right while I had things to do, but when I ran out of things to do I got a bit cheesed off with the whole thing.'
- 'I felt fed up, frustrated. What do you do?'
- 'Why did the whole family come? Whose was the problem – the child's or the family's?'

Group's feelings

The GP's frustration seemed to be related to the power there is in silence. Is there a power struggle in trying to get the patient to talk? Silence from Anne makes both the mother and the GP anxious. The mother is determined that the girl needs help. Is this a way of getting the mother's attention and involvement?

The doctor feels that 'something must be done'. Is this coming from the child or the family? There seems to be an element of competition as to who has the worst illness in the family. The situation remained unresolved because Anne would not do what is expected of every patient – that is, reveal her problem. The group felt angry, but they also felt guilty about being angry because this was a very sick family. It was suggested that Anne wanted the whole family in the room to demonstrate their problems to the GP. The family seemed to express every emotion except anger.

The presenter said 'Anne has a lot of reasons to be stressed. Nevertheless, just sitting there and bawling her eyes out is not going to achieve anything. In many ways, it is typical of adolescence!'

Themes

- There is a need for the GP to 'do something'.
- Non-verbal communication is powerful.
- Diagnosing the cause of the problem can be difficult and frustrating.
- The adolescent is part of a family with associated dynamics.
- Families and adolescents who seem to be unable to take action to solve their problem put further pressure on the GP to 'do something'.
- The adolescent is brought by a parent rather than making her own appointment.
- The parent does the talking.
- Multiple health professionals are involved, which can lead to difficulties.
- The GP is tempted to take on a parental role and to feel responsible – to have to cure the problem herself.

Overriding emotions

- Presenter: concerned, frustrated, anxious, angry, helpless, uneasy.
- Group: empathy, anger, irritation, guilt, sadness.

Group leader's comments

The main problem in this case seems to have been in establishing an effective doctor–patient relationship in order to make a diagnosis. The GP, the practice nurse and the group were overwhelmed. Was this due to the parents' serious medical problems? Did this reflect how Anne felt? The need to 'do something' reduced the ability of both the doctor and the group to empathise with the patient herself, rather than with her family as a whole. The GP felt that she was under pressure and argued that she found herself in an impossible position. No wonder she felt that she had to refer the patient – to the nurse and then to the child psychiatrist – and she also felt the need to initiate the prescription for antidepressants. How helpful were these measures? What was the effect on the doctor–patient relationship?

Chapter 3

Organising the material

This chapter is for the benefit of future researchers who may be interested in the practical problems that we faced in carrying out this research project. Readers who are more interested in the consultations may wish to turn straight to Part 2.

Notes on methodology

Definition of 'a consultation'

During the first presentation (*see* Case A on page 6) it became clear that we had not accurately defined 'a consultation'. Some group members assumed that this would be a single contact with a health professional. Others, like the presenter in Case A, felt that it was necessary to present a developing story of multiple contacts in order to demonstrate the complexity of the interaction. After discussion it was agreed that each presenter would choose what was appropriate for him- or herself.

Reviewing the cases

Identifying the doctor's feelings and the group's feelings

The group focused its attention on the mixture of events and feelings that were presented and which prompted the presenter to select a particular consultation to share with the group. It had been agreed that we would record the doctor's feelings and the subsequent feelings engendered in the group.

Identifying themes

The groups sought to identify the difficulties within the consultation that had caused problems for the presenter. Our aim here was to identify these difficulties, which we believe are likely to be present in other adolescent consultations and which, if understood, might prevent future difficulties from occurring in contacts with other young people. It was hoped that, by being aware of these difficulties, professionals would be able to alter their behaviour within the doctor–patient interaction and so avoid future pitfalls.

The work of the editorial team

After the six Balint meetings, a group of four (the two group leaders, the healthcare researcher and the child/adolescent psychiatrist) undertook the task of writing up the material.

The themes and emotions identified by the group were used as titles to summarise the cases in table format. This enabled common themes to be looked for across all cases. By systematically studying all of the cases, it became more apparent that themes discussed in later cases were also relevant to those presented in earlier meetings. In addition to those themes that were summarised by the group in the last session, some further themes were identified when reading the case transcripts. Short vignettes were produced to enable quick reference to the cases. These are presented in Appendix 4.

Part 2 of this book gives an account of each case presentation, followed by notes on the doctor's feelings, the group's feelings, themes, and comments from the group leader.

In Part 3 we discuss factors that may affect consultations with adolescents. These include the role of parents, the structure of the NHS, the confusion over where responsibility lies, the doctor's feelings, the developmental process of adolescence, and adolescents' views of primary care.

Part 4 gives the personal perspectives of a GP, a practice nurse, a child/adolescent psychiatrist, and a ChildLine worker.

Finance

At the start of the project there were no financial resources. Later a grant was secured from the Omega Foundation (*see* page x). This enabled a small payment to be made to members of the editorial team for the time they gave to writing this book, and also to those who made a contribution to Part 4.

Part 2

The case presentations

Chapter 1

Case 1: 'Mary' – should we look for hidden agendas?

Presenter:	GP: female, white, British.
Patient:	Mary: 16 years old, female, white, British.
Setting:	One visit to the GP surgery.

What happened

- *One contact: Mary visits the GP surgery.*
  Mary opens the conversation:
  Mary: 'I have acne. My mum says there is a pill I can take which is good for it.'
  GP: 'There is a pill for acne. Why do you think your mother has suggested it?'
  Mary: 'I have a boyfriend.'
  GP: 'Do you think your mother wants you to be a little safer?'
  Mary: No reply.
  GP: 'Have you had intercourse?'
  Mary: 'Someone forced me into it.' She looks embarrassed.
  The GP said that as the acne was not bad she gave Mary a choice of three things – topical or oral antibiotics, or the pill.

  The GP added that, as Mary was working, the cost of the prescription concerned her, so she chose the pill because she did not have to pay for it. The GP continued, 'We talked about whether she wanted to have sex or not. I said she didn't have to and that it was her choice. She didn't say much. I did most of the talking, saying my standard piece when prescribing the pill. She seemed a little awkward about it, and I got the impression that it was at her mother's suggestion rather than something she cared about.' The GP concluded 'We talked about smoking – they all smoke. I told her she must stop, and that was that. Fairly standard sort of request and consultation.'

Doctor's feelings

'I felt like I usually do in these situations: Uuuh! It's like a routine. I tend to go through the same sorts of things. My heart goes out to them. Because they are progressing almost too rapidly for themselves. They obviously feel they ought to be "doing it", but I am not sure they want to.'

Group's feelings

The group recognised from their own experience the conflict felt by this GP. Her counter-transference expressed in the phrase 'My heart goes out to them' does not make her feel at ease in the medical role she has to play. Moreover, although she says the decision about whether to have sex must be that of the patient, when she says 'They are progressing almost too rapidly for themselves' she implies that developmentally this may be difficult for Mary. 'After all, Mary is still getting her mother to do the requesting, even if she is not present in the consultation. How much is the mother actually involved?'

There is a further problem for the GP. To what extent should she be looking behind the request for a hidden agenda? Maybe the acne and a cheap prescription are all that there is to this consultation.

The group felt that there were times when GPs saw sexually active behaviour behind every female adolescent consultation. This can embarrass many 15- to 17-year-olds and even put pressure on them to start before they are ready. However, for those who are sexually active and not on contraception it is important for the GP to help the adolescent to reveal the situation. One person suggested that it may be easier to ask directly for contraception at a family planning clinic, whereas at a general practice one needed a 'presenting ticket'.

Members of the group questioned how the consultation might have gone if the girl had seen a male GP, and whether she would have been inhibited about discussing sex and possibly left with a cream for her acne instead. The group felt that the personality of the GP was most important, but that gender, age and ethnicity may also impact on the adolescent's willingness to disclose their full agenda.

Themes

- Is sex behind many female adolescent consultations?
- Should the GP probe in order to find out?
- The mother, even if not present, plays a part in the consultations.
- Some GPs feel a conflict between their professional role and a protective parental role.
- The gender of the GP and the adolescent may play a role. Would it be more difficult for a girl to discuss contraception with a male doctor?

Overriding emotions

- Presenter: sympathetic towards the girl, frustrated, parental.
- Group: sympathy for the girl, uncertainty.

Group leader's comments

In this case the GP assumed, probably correctly, that there was a hidden agenda, but something prevented her from taking up the patient's cue 'Someone forced me into it' (meaning sexual intercourse). The doctor reverted to her 'standard piece'. Was this a defence? She began to generalise – for example, saying 'They all smoke' – and the group colluded. No one challenged her. In a Balint group, generalisations suggest that something is being avoided and I, as the leader, failed to address this, too. Were we all afraid of opening Pandora's box, or was this an example of our inability to hear what was being said?

Chapter 2

Case 2: 'Harold' – aggression

Presenter:	GP: female, black.
Patient:	Harold: 13 years old, male, black, West Indian. Moved to London from the Caribbean at the age of 11 years.
Setting:	Several visits to the GP surgery.

What happened

- *Contacts: the GP saw Harold with his mother on several occasions at the GP surgery.*
  Harold was a 13-year-old West Indian boy. When he was 7 years old his parents emigrated to England, leaving him in the West Indies with his grandparents. When he was 11 years old his mother, hearing something that made her feel worried about how he was being treated, summoned him to London. In England he was met by his mother, with a new stepfather and a two-and-a-half year old stepsister whom he knew nothing about. Harold hated his stepfather. However, he did see something of his father who lived nearby.

  Harold had difficulty settling into his new school. He was excluded on two occasions for chasing the girls. There was a vague story of him attempting to touch their breasts. After a few weeks the school took him back.

  His behaviour did not improve. Before seeing the GP he had been excluded for the third time. On this occasion he also hit his teacher. The school told his mother that they would not take him back until the whole family had been 'sorted out' by the GP.

  The GP said that she had rung the school to talk to someone about what Harold had done, but no one seemed able or willing to help her.

  After seeing Harold and his mother on a few occasions, she came to the conclusion that the family dynamics and Harold's aggressive, possibly sexual behaviour needed more skilled treatment than she could provide. She rang the Child and Adolescent Department and found out to her dismay that it would be at least three months before he could be seen, even as an urgent appointment.

Doctor's feelings

The presenting doctor said that she rather liked Harold, especially when he said 'I didn't hit the teacher as hard as I could have.'

She felt concerned about leaving Harold unhappy at home and excluded from school. She felt that he would be likely to roam the streets and get into more trouble.

'I felt that a problem that was too big for me had been dumped on me, and others did not wish to help sort it out. The school had washed their hands of him, the parents were part of the problem, and back-up services were not available for some time.'

She felt that Harold's aggressive and possibly sexual behaviour was difficult to accept in a British school, whereas the situation might have been different in his home environment in the West Indies.

She wondered if he had experienced racist bullying. The GP was black and she felt that, because of her colour, Harold was at ease with her. However, she said 'I did not want to get involved. The problem was too big. And I would be leaving the practice in three months' time.'

Group's feelings

The group recognised that problems were dumped on GPs and that they could not refuse a case as other services could.

The group felt frustrated with the system – that the school would not help and the psychiatric services were overloaded.

Members of the group questioned whether behaviour that is considered inappropriate in the UK might have been more acceptable when Harold was with his grandparents in the Caribbean.

Although Harold's behaviour at school conjures up an image of an aggressive adolescent, the group warmed to him and were 'on his side'.

The group was concerned about all the changes that Harold was facing – having to adjust to a different culture as well as a different family structure at the time of early adolescence.

Themes

- Young men may have difficulties discussing sexual and aggressive feelings.
- GPs may find it difficult to discuss sexual and aggressive feelings with young men.
- Problems which are too difficult for others to 'sort out' may be dumped on GPs.
- Back-up services, such as those provided by psychiatric units, are often not available for months.
- What is acceptable behaviour during adolescence in our culture?
- GPs may find it difficult to discuss issues that touch on an unresolved problem in their own youth.
- The gender of the GP and the adolescent may play a role.
- Young black men may find it easier to relate to black doctors.
- The building and sustaining of a relationship are undermined by lack of continuity of care.
- The adolescent is brought to see the GP by a parent.

Overriding emotions

- Presenter: frustrated, angry, put upon, not wanting to get involved, unsupported.
- Group: sympathy for the GP, frustration.

Group leader's comments

It was clear that the doctor and patient had a good relationship, but the doctor felt out of her depth, particularly as her time at the practice was so limited. The group identified the need for the patient to be supported at a time when there were many changes occurring, both in himself and in his circumstances. Perhaps an effective partnership between the practice and support services was what was required, but this is now often lacking, leaving the GP and patient in difficulty.

Chapter 3

Case 3: 'Richard' – depression

Presenter:	GP: female, white.
Patient:	Richard: 16 years old, male, white, British.
Setting:	Five contacts at the GP surgery (two with the practice nurse and three with the GP).

What happened

- *Contact 1: his mother brings Richard to see the practice nurse.*
  His mother brought 16-year-old Richard to see the practice nurse. She said that her son was suffering from insomnia, had been aggressive towards her and his younger sister, was not getting up for college in the morning, was not tidying his room and was arguing a lot. The nurse referred the boy to the GP.
- *Contact 2: Richard visits the GP with his mother.*
  Richard lives with his mother and his three sisters. Their mother brought them up, as the father has not been around much and has another family. The mother asked Richard's father to talk to the boy when he started having difficulties, but the father was not interested. The mother expressed difficulty in raising a son, which she saw as different to raising daughters. One of Richard's older sisters became pregnant as a teenager and had a baby three years ago. The family lives in a small village for which the bus service has been discontinued. This makes it difficult for the boy to meet up with other young people, as he has no friends in the village.
- *For the next part of the consultation the GP saw Richard alone.*
  Richard complained of difficulty in sleeping since he had taken his GCSEs the previous summer. He went to sleep at 2a.m. and woke at 8a.m., and he felt tired during the day. During the course of the summer holidays this situation had improved. After returning to college he felt worried and reduced his workload to relieve his stress. He said that he did not use drugs. The GP felt that he might be depressed, and gave him a leaflet on depression and a directory of services for young people which included a freephone line, the addresses of counsellors, and information on sexual health services.
- *Contact 3: Richard returns to see the practice nurse with his mother.*
  Richard's mother complained that they were arguing because Richard would not get up in the morning for college. He felt that he could not manage the work, but his mother felt he was capable. The nurse suggested to his mother some strategies for avoiding conflict.
- *Contact 4: Richard visits the GP with his mother.*

Richard and his mother agreed that he has symptoms of depression, including low mood, low self-esteem, poor sleep, poor appetite and loss of interest. The GP prescribed lofepramine and referred him to the local child and adolescent psychiatrist. During the consultation the boy was co-operative. He and his mother disagreed about his level of aggression and his sister's contribution to his fights with her. Richard was reasonably easy to talk to, and his mother allowed him to talk. He did not see his aggression as a problem.

- Contact 5: Richard visits the GP alone for a follow-up appointment.
  Richard was feeling better and was back at college. His mother was leaving it up to him to tidy his room, and they were arguing less. His mother has not been in contact with the surgery again.

Doctor's feelings

The GP felt that Richard was not very keen to open up and he responded better to direct questions. She felt that with adolescents one needed to think about the questions to ask, and to ask them 'in the right way', particularly with boys.

The GP felt that the absence of the father was significant, although Richard said that he did not care. She felt that the boy might be lacking a male role model, which may have led to his difficulties in managing aggression. The GP felt she was yet another female involved with the boy, and that he might have benefited from seeing a male GP. However, once he had started with her it was difficult to transfer him because they had already established a relationship.

She felt that the boy did not come over very well. He 'did not have much personality', but she still liked him. She felt that he communicated a lot non-verbally. He did take part when he was there with his mother, which seemed healthy. He had respect for his mother, who had made an attempt to deal with the problem and had come up with one or two solutions. He had also come on his own, negotiated when he would like to come back again, and given consent for the GP to share the information. The GP felt that this 'said a lot'.

Group's feelings

One member of the group felt that the consultation seemed smooth, and was puzzled that the mother described an aggressive boy when in fact he came passively. Another group member felt surprised that he was so willing to come. It was felt that he came as a small child without protest and sounded very amenable.

The group questioned whether he would go to the child psychiatrist, and whether he would go alone or with his mother. It was felt that he acknowledged there was something in him that was not right, or he would not have come.

The group wondered about his sexual development. There was the feeling that something was going on that could not be seen. Could Richard be worried over his changing body, his developing aggressive and sexual (possibly homosexual) feelings and that there was no male in the family with whom to share his concerns?

The group discussed the gender of the GP. Would the boy have chosen to see a female GP? Would topics such as masturbation be difficult for him or the GP to discuss? It was suggested that he might be offered the opportunity to see a male GP in the practice, although it was acknowledged that he might already have some attachment to this GP and might not want to lose this. Would he have the opportunity to see a male psychiatrist?

He may come back because he wants to say something but cannot quite articulate it. He may be doing badly at college, he may feel he is homosexual, may be worried about things that are going on at home, or he may be angry with his father. We do not know, and we have to tolerate not knowing.

The 'room-tidying' conflict was regarded as a common one. It was defined as a problem by the mother but not by the boy. His mother had chosen to bring this issue and the discussion about aggression into the surgery, whereas others might not have done.

Some members of the group felt that the boy was not giving as much as he could, and that the consultation was intellectual rather than emotional. This seemed to be reflected in the group response, which appeared to be lacking in emotion and flat. One group member wondered if Richard was in fact repressed rather than depressed, and if he might be ashamed of his feelings. Was there some shame for him in experiencing adolescence as a man? He might be feeling bad about himself, or have low self-esteem. Or he might not want to share his feelings, and might feel that he ought to be good like his little sister. Was he experiencing anxiety that was not being recognised? One group member mentioned recent press reports of under-achievement by boys within society and education.

Some group members felt frustrated that there was something difficult to get to, while others felt some optimism. Since the boy had come back to the surgery, the intervention seemed to be working in a positive way. The GP was congratulated on getting on with the problem while psychiatric services had not been helpful.

Themes

- Boys find it hard to understand let alone talk about their feelings.
- Is it unreasonable for GPs to expect teenage boys to describe this private world verbally? Is developing a private world which is not shared with adults part of adolescence?
- What is acceptable behaviour in adolescence? Is room-tidying an appropriate problem to bring to the GP?
- We have to tolerate not knowing the whole picture.
- The gender of the GP and adolescent may play a role. Is it more difficult for a male adolescent to talk to a female doctor about masturbation and homosexuality?
- Boys whose divorced fathers appear to neglect them are deprived of an important aspect of male self-esteem. Is it important for them to be seen by a male professional?
- 'Something must be done.'
- The adolescent was brought to see the GP by his parent.

Overriding emotions

- Presenter: impatient, annoyed, frustrated, angry, agitated, 'adolescent', relieved.
- Group: sympathy with the presenter, curiosity.

Group leader's comments

In this case the group congratulated the GP on 'getting on with the problem' while 'the psychiatric services had not been helpful'. The doctor felt that the patient was not keen to open up but 'responded to direct questions', and that 'he did not have much personality'. Similarly, it was observed that the consultations and the group discussion were lacking in emotion. There seemed to be a reluctance on all sides to 'get involved'. Is that why the doctor was congratulated? Is that why the patient was referred and given antidepressants?

Chapter 4

Case 4: 'Ann' – getting it right

Presenter:	GP: female, white, British.
Patient:	Ann: 12 years old, female, white, British.
Setting:	Two visits to the GP surgery.

What happened

- *Contact 1: Ann's mother brings her to see the GP for an emergency appointment.*
  The GP has known Ann all her life. The GP began, 'It was at the end of a particularly horrible Monday morning surgery. When I saw her name on the list I thought "Uuuh!".' This was because of past problems when the patient had hurt herself at school and the GP had had to deal with a 'great fuss' and had finally referred her to the child psychiatrist.
  'In came Ann. She was quiet and rather thin. I thought "Is she anorexic?"'
  Her mother said 'I have brought her along because she won't go to school and she is ill, and at school they say she can't be ill all this time and we have got to do something about it!'

GP:	'Are you not feeling well?'
Ann:	'No, I don't feel well.'
GP:	'In what way don't you feel well?'
Mother:	'She doesn't eat anything and I think she is anaemic. She has got a terrible sore throat. She's always got a sore throat. I couldn't come every time she had a sore throat or we would be living in your surgery.'
GP:	'How is your throat today?'
Ann:	'Sore.'

The GP felt Ann's neck but could not find any glands. She looked down her throat without a spatula. It was a little red. The GP thought 'I am going to keep this physical.'

GP:	'I'll take a throat swab and if it does not grow anything we will do a blood test to see if you have glandular fever.'

The mother looked quite pleased at this. So the GP got her throat swab.

GP:	'Would you please open your mouth.'
Ann:	'No, I'm not having it done' (like a two-year-old).

Ann's mother desperately tried to persuade her to have it done, but Ann was adamant. The GP thought 'This is all I need.'

GP: 'It's entirely up to you' (thinking 'If you want it, have it. If you do not, I am not going to have a power struggle with you').

Mother: 'If you don't have it, Ann, you'll have to have a blood test.'

Ann: 'All right.'

The GP told the group 'Fortunately the blood collection had gone, so I pointed out that she would have to go to the hospital. I filled in the form and told her to come back and see me in a week.'

- *Contact 2: mother and Ann visit the GP.*

'To my amazement they both came back to see me by appointment the following week. Ann had been for the blood test and the result was normal. I was calmer and we had a reasonable conversation about why Ann feared returning to school and about her fears of eating, which seemed to be related to an obsessional fear of contracting an infection.'

Doctor's feelings

'I felt more and more agitated. I felt I was going into "adolescent mode". I thought, "Here I am, at 58, producing an adolescent response." I was thinking, "I must not react like this." However, I wanted to shake her.'

Later she felt very angry with herself. 'When she had gone I felt terrible. I was furious and could kick myself because it came home to me just what had happened in this consultation.' She felt that she had behaved really badly, that Ann would not come back to see her, and that there would probably be another 'big fuss'. She was relieved when the girl did return and she had a chance to amend the situation.

Group's feelings

The group raised questions about the girl's behaviour. Was there a physical problem, an eating disorder, or a problem at school or at home?

The group felt that there was often a self-imposed pressure making conscientious GPs believe that it is vitally important when seeing teenagers 'to get it right'. There is a belief that if the doctor 'got it wrong' they would somehow ruin that young person's attitude to general practice for years to come. This has something to do with a feeling of omnipotence – that is, that what GPs do is of overwhelming importance – whereas it is just one of many adult reactions which the teenager will experience.

The need to 'get it right' amplifies other aspects of the doctor experience with regard to the consultation. In this case previous knowledge of the patient coloured the GP's approach and attitude to the patient, and may have influenced the course and outcome of the consultation.

Themes

- The need to 'get it right', and the belief that if the doctor 'got it wrong' they would somehow ruin that young person's attitude to general practice for years to come.
- The feeling of omnipotence of the GP, which may be present in many consultations with adolescents.
- The mother and school demanding of the GP that 'something must be done'.
- The adolescent is brought to see the GP by a parent.
- In the consultation the mother does much of the talking.
- Non-verbal communication is significant, with the girl sitting with her mouth shut.
- The arousal of anger and frustration in the doctor by 'non-cooperation' of the adolescent.
- Time pressure of emergency appointments at the end of surgery can influence attitudes to the patient.
- Knowing a patient well can affect a consultation, and not necessarily in a positive way.

Overriding emotions

- Presenter: impatient, annoyed, frustrated, angry, agitated, 'adolescent', relieved.
- Group: sympathy with the presenter, curiosity.

Group leader's comments

In this case the doctor lost her professional identity because of the parental and adolescent feelings which the patient engendered in her. The need to 'get it right' interfered with her ability to identify the patient's real problem. However, the doctor's emotional response demonstrated to the patient that she cared. Was this why Ann felt able to come back? Did she recognise that the doctor was 'there' for her? The doctor felt that she was fortunate to be given a second chance.

Although the doctor's feeling of omnipotence was recognised, the group was able to point out that this episode reflected just one of many adult reactions which the adolescent will experience.

Chapter 5

Case 5: 'Sally' – confidentiality

Cases 5 and 6 highlight the importance and impact of maintaining confidentiality in adolescent consultations.

Presenter:	Psychiatrist: female, white, South African.
Patient:	Sally: 16 years old, female, white, British.
Setting:	Several visits to the psychiatrist at the Child Psychiatry Unit.

What happened

- *Contacts: several consultations on a weekly basis over a period of months.*
  An adolescent psychiatrist in the group discussed a girl whom she had seen after she had been admitted to hospital having taken an overdose. She saw the girl on a weekly basis for a few months and developed a good relationship with her. The girl was experiencing difficulties with her relationship with her parents, but refused to allow involvement of her parents in her treatment.

  The psychiatrist was to leave the clinic in three months' time, and she wished to transfer her patient on to a colleague. However, when she asked the patient's permission to tell the colleague about her problems, permission was denied and the patient refused to see anyone else. She agreed that her GP could be informed that she had received treatment, without details of the content being disclosed.

  Confidentiality was preserved, but the psychiatrist carried some anxieties when she left her patient unsupported. The doctor thought that Sally was no longer suffering from depression and had no suicidal thoughts, but she felt that she remained generally vulnerable.

Doctor's feelings

The psychiatrist was concerned for the girl. She felt torn between the need to respect Sally's right to confidentiality and her wish to make sure that she received follow-on care. Although she felt that the girl was able to make her own decision, the psychiatrist still felt responsible for her well-being and was anxious about leaving her. The psychiatrist was left with a burden of anxiety.

Group's feelings

- Concern for the girl.
- Empathy with the psychiatrist.
- Maintaining confidentiality is very important, but it can make life difficult for the professional.

Themes

- The decision not to break confidentiality may leave the doctor carrying a burden of uncertainty and worry.
- Confidentiality is important, but absolute confidentiality cannot always be guaranteed. An 'escape clause' needs to be included.
- Suicidal intent is a situation where the commitment to confidentiality might be broken in the patient's interest, because of the threat of possible harm to the patient. Handling these situations can be difficult.

Overriding emotions

- Group: anxiety about the safety of the patient, conflict regarding when to break confidentiality.

Group leader's comments

This doctor was presented with a difficult dilemma. The case emphasises the need for those working with adolescents to be able to cope with uncertainty and anxiety. The group appreciated the considerable cost to the doctor of maintaining her patient's confidentiality.

Chapter 6

Case 6: 'Gita' – confidentiality

Presenter:	Health promotion nurse: female, white.
Patient:	Gita: 14 years old, female, Asian.
Setting:	Teen clinic at the GP surgery.

What happened

This case was reported second-hand by a group member who was involved in helping a practice to set up a teen clinic. The clinic was set up by a practice nurse and health visitor.

The clinic's third patient was a 14-year-old Hindu girl. She asked about confidentiality and was assured that whatever information she shared in the clinic would not get back to her family.

She then disclosed that she was being sexually abused at home. This caused considerable upset to the organisers of the clinic, who found it difficult to handle the situation.

Eventually they shared the information with the GP, and the girl gave them permission to refer her to a team more used to handling this problem.

Nurse's feelings

The professional who was running the clinic felt unprepared to handle this case. They wanted to respect confidentiality but needed support, and initially they were not clear about child protection issues. Once the girl had given permission to be referred, all of them were relieved.

Group's feelings

- Concern for the girl and sympathy for the team who had such a difficult case early on in the life of the teen clinic.
- Maintaining confidentiality is very important, but it can be difficult for the professionals.
- It is important to have a 'get-out' clause in confidentiality statements to cover issues such as sexual abuse and suicidal intent.

Themes

- Confidentiality is important, but absolute confidentiality cannot always be guaranteed. An 'escape clause' needs to be included.
- It is important to convey the policy on confidentiality to teenagers. It should be available in written form, and stated verbally in the consultation.
- If a parent is involved but not present, it helps if the doctor and patient agree before the end of the consultation what, if anything, is to be passed on.
- Sexual abuse is a situation where the commitment to confidentiality might be broken in the patient's interest, because of the threat of harm to the patient or others in the family. Handling these situations can be difficult. *See* Appendix 3.
- If adolescents are encouraged to share their problems, such cases will arise and teams need to be prepared to deal with them.

Overriding emotions

- Group: anxiety about the safety of the patient, conflict regarding when to break confidentiality.

Group leader's comments

This situation was unusual, especially for a Balint group, as the presenter was not directly involved in the case. The group appreciated that this case emphasises the need for clarity and explanation of exceptions when assuring confidentiality. This case also illustrates the problems that can occur when difficulties such as those relating to child protection issues have not been foreseen.

Chapter 7

Case 7: 'Fatima' – a question of culture?

Presenter:	GP: female, Asian.
Patient:	Fatima: 16 years old, female, Asian/British.
Setting:	Two visits to the GP at the university practice, and one meeting in the street.

What happened

- *Contact 1: Fatima visits the university practice surgery.*
  'This is a 16-year-old Asian girl. She came to see me at the beginning of the autumn school term. The counsellor at the school had asked her to see a doctor because she was worried about her physical condition. She was thin and not eating well.'

  She was articulate and was working hard for her 'A'-levels. At the end of the previous term her family had discovered that she had a boyfriend and had 'gone mad about it'. She had been living with her mother and older brother at the time. Her father had died previously and this brother was now head of the family. Fatima described her family as very controlling and as emotionally abusing her.

  She was very angry with her family – so much so that she moved out to live with her other brother and his wife. This brother is 'schizophrenic', but in the family's culture mental illness is taboo. Therefore they pretend that the brother's illness does not exist (another example of denial).

  'The first time I saw her I felt this arrangement was OK. She was seeing the counsellor at school and found this very helpful. I checked her physically and talked about how I could help her. She felt things were contained.'
- *Contact 2: Fatima visits the practice again.*
  A few weeks later Fatima returned to the surgery. The situation in the brother's home had deteriorated, and she felt that she was being emotionally abused and belittled. She was expected to conform to what her family expected of her, and they would not even cook for her. She was agitated and angry, and she felt that she had to stay in her room.

  'We discussed what I could do for her. She did not want social services involved. She wanted to remain where she was – or preferably move in with her other uncle. However, she knew this was unacceptable, as he was unmarried.'

  'She felt things could just about be contained. She was not depressed. She did not have an eating disorder. Her periods were OK. I felt she was vulnerable but did not know how to help her. I asked her about physical violence, but not sexual abuse. It did not cross my mind.'

- *Contact 3: a meeting in the street.*
  The brother had been admitted to hospital because of his schizophrenia, and Fatima was on the way back from visiting him. She seemed OK. The GP asked her to come for another appointment, but she has not done so.

Doctor's feelings

- 'I liked her. I liked her spirit.'
- Anxious because she does not know the community and is not part of the culture.
- Unsure about whether she should get involved or leave the case to the school counsellor.
- Concerned because she did not know what happened next, and felt that it was left unresolved. 'I have worried about her a lot – but maybe she wasn't coming to ask me to help with those problems. Maybe it is more my anxiety about the situation.'

Group's feelings

The group discussion centred on this girl's religion. One Asian GP felt that some girls' lives could be in danger when they stray from the values of their parents' community. 'Some families find the shame so great they would even consider killing their daughters.' It was thought that religious leaders would be more likely to side with the family. Although reacting against her family, Fatima identified with the Asian culture. She described herself as Asian, and her boyfriend is Asian. 'I am not having sex because I am an Asian girl.' One member of the group pointed out that Asian girls are expected to be successful academically but to toe the line socially. They may see education as a way to escape.

One group member thought that the GP was being educated by the patient. Another felt that the girl was manipulating the GP. Most of the group were concerned about the girl. One question summed this up: 'Would you take steps to check what is happening to her?' The GP answered 'If she didn't have a counsellor at school I would have been more worried, and perhaps would have tried to get her to come back on a regular basis.'

The group found it hard to establish what was the responsibility of the GP. This reflected the central problem that maintained the GP's anxiety and prompted her to share this case. 'A 16-year-old in trouble and another doctor asked me to check her physically. Hearing her problem, my parental feelings became active – I felt it must be up to me to help this girl.' Professionally the GP let the patient carry the responsibility herself – she respected the girl's autonomy, but continued to worry.

Themes

- Problems arise from living in two cultures.
- There is a problem of understanding and respecting other people's cultural values when your patient is from a different culture.

- Whose responsibility is it to cope with these problems? It is that of the girl, the counsellor, the GP or the family?
- If young people do not come back, should the GP contact them?
- The need is felt to protect the girl, to take her side – yet we do not know the whole picture.
- Conflict within the family is often presented to the GP.
- A feeling of omnipotence in the GP.

Overriding emotions

- Presenter: concerned, anxious, frustrated, impotent.
- Group: concerned, frustrated, feeling of being manipulated.

Group leader's comments

The doctor may have underestimated the value to the patient of having a doctor who listened attentively. Some of the frustration and discomfort in the group may reflect the difficulty in understanding different cultures and recognising our own prejudices. Perhaps a more open discussion would have been helpful.

Chapter 8

Case 8: 'Mary' – whose responsibility?

Presenter:	GP/consultant: male, white, British.
Patient:	Mary: 18 years old, female, white, British.
Setting:	Routine follow-up appointment with consultant at an oncology clinic.

What happened

- *Contact 1: Mary visits the paediatric cancer outpatient clinic with her mother.*
  During the consultation Mary sat looking at the floor. Her mother told her story.

  Mother: 'When 11 years old Mary was admitted to hospital with lymphoma. She hated being the eldest on the children's ward, the cytotoxic drugs and the loss of hair. A large mass was removed from her abdomen. She fought through all this and recovered. When Mary returned home, her mother took her to the local secondary school. She was shown around by the headmistress who was very pleasant. Two weeks later, she received a letter refusing her a place because of the health record.'

  Doctor: 'That's outrageous!'

  Mother: 'We appealed and the school's decision was overturned.'

Mary has now left school and has been seeking employment. She was shortlisted for three posts, and she felt that all of the interviews went well, but she was not offered any of the jobs. She feels there is no point continuing the search, as no one will accept her because of her cancer history.

The doctor examined Mary and, as expected, found her physically fit. He was now convinced that Mary was damaged psychologically, but what could he do to restore her self-esteem?

He offered to provide a letter from the hospital saying that she was fit and had little chance of having a recurrence seven years after treatment. 'I felt sad as she left, and a failure at not helping her more.'

Doctor's feelings

The doctor described his anger and his desire to go out and fight against this new form of discrimination. These were out-of-date attitudes! After all she had been through, Mary deserved better than this, especially now that her chances of a recurrence so many years after treatment were no higher than those of her contemporaries.

Group's feelings

The group empathised with the doctor. They felt sorry for the girl and angry about the discrimination. However, as the discussion continued, the group questioned whether it really was Mary's risk of cancer that was putting off potential employers. If her subdued interactions during the consultation were repeated in an interview situation, this might have deterred the employers. The group then felt that it was perhaps more important to tackle her self-esteem. They had taken on the girl's perceptions without stepping back or questioning them.

Themes

- Whose responsibility is it to cope with these problems? Is it that of the girl, the family, or the doctor?
- If the doctor takes on responsibility for issues he or she cannot resolve, he or she is doomed to failure. However if the doctor works with the patient, encouraging them to take on responsibility, he or she is likely to be more effective.
- When a doctor's paternalistic feelings are aroused, it is hard not to feel that the task is to protect and fight for his or her young patients.
- Sympathy for the patient may cloud the doctor's objectivity.

Overriding emotions

- Presenter: protective, angry, furious at the injustice, impotent.
- Group: concern for the doctor, annoyance with the school, anger at the injustice, frustration with the girl.

Postscript

- *At Mary's next appointment, six months later, after the case had been presented to the group.* Mary spoke this time: 'I'm going to be a taxi driver.' Her uncle had given her a Vespa. With a friend who was also training, she had already visited many parts of London and was learning the streets. 'I'll work on my own, I won't need others to employ me.' She seemed determined and enthusiastic.

Doctor's feelings

'My anger set me off believing I should fight on Mary's behalf. I did not see that she was capable of coping and that it was her responsibility, not mine. I failed to see her "positive side", that had brought her through her cancer. I had labelled her a victim, rather than encouraging her to find her own solution.'

'After the first consultation I felt I had let her down. After seeing her again I felt full of admiration for her finding a practical solution to her problem.'

Group leader's comments

The doctor became angry about the discrimination against his patient: 'That's outrageous.' Did this anger and frustration come from the patient? The group recognised that this reaction may have clouded the doctor's objectivity. However, the postscript (which occurred after the ending of the group and therefore could not be discussed) demonstrates that the doctor might have helped to empower his patient to find a solution for herself with the support of her family.

Case 9: 'Aisa' – failure of the system

Presenter:	GP: female, Asian.
Patient:	Aisa: 18 years old, female, Asian.
Setting:	Several visits to the university practice: two visits to the practice nurse, three visits to the GP (one at an emergency clinic), one visit to another GP partner, two calls to the out-of-hours service, one visit to the family GP, and one phone call from the GP.

What happened

- *Contact 1: Aisa visits the practice nurse at the university practice surgery, alone.*
  'Aisa, a first-year undergraduate aged 18 years, came to the practice nurse for a health check. Vaginal thrush was diagnosed and Canesten prescribed.'
- *Contact 2: Aisa visits the practice nurse at the university practice surgery, alone.*
  Aisa returned with a recurrence a few weeks later and was given more Canesten.
- *Contact 3: Aisa attends an emergency clinic at the university practice surgery, alone.*
  Aisa saw the doctor at an emergency clinic with another recurrence of her vaginal symptoms. 'I gave her more Canesten and suggested she made an appointment for a vaginal examination'. Aisa then mentioned that she was wondering whether she should go on the pill. 'I gave her a pamphlet to read.'
- *Contact 4: Aisa visits the GP presenter at the university practice surgery, alone.*
  'She kept her appointment with me. A cracked vulva, typical of thrush, was revealed at the examination. I took swabs and prescribed more Canesten.' Aisa said she was in a hurry to get to a lecture, so did not wish to discuss contraception at that time.
- *Contact 5: Aisa visits another GP at the university practice surgery, alone.*
  'This was one of my partners. He started Aisa on the pill and gave her more Canesten.'
- *Contact 6: Aisa again visits the GP presenter at the university practice surgery, alone.*
  'When I saw her yet again I noticed the swab was negative.' Aisa said that the symptoms had cleared and mentioned she had had unprotected sex with her boyfriend. 'At this point alarm bells should have rung, but they didn't.'
  The presenting doctor did not see her again.
- *Contact 7: home visit by 'out-of-hours' service, with a friend in the room.*
  The out-of-hours service visited Aisa at the weekend. She was having a panic attack and

was hyperventilating. She had a friend in her room and did not want to talk, but intimated that she had seen her family GP and was on antibiotics for pelvic inflammation.
- *Contact 8: home visit by 'out-of-hours' service, alone.*
  The out-of-hours service visited Aisa again because of sickness caused by pregnancy.
- *Contact 9: telephone call from the GP.*
  The presenting doctor rang Aisa to ask what was happening about the pregnancy. Aisa said that she had been to the family planning clinic and had been referred for termination. She added in an angry way 'Oh, it wasn't thrush.'

Doctor's feelings

The doctor felt that the dates suggested Aisa had been pregnant when she first came to see her. 'I felt that I and the practice let her down, perhaps because Aisa had behaved in an adolescent way.'

When pushed, she added 'She made me feel like a frustrated parent. Aisa was not willing to play by adult rules and not willing to tell me the whole story.'

'Because I am seen as an authority figure and fellow Asian, some students may find it difficult to talk to me. Some feel it might get back to their parents.'

'I have seen a lot of Asian patients. This patient struck me as fairly confident. She was a very attractive, very pretty girl. I would actually say she wilfully misled us, as if she really did not want us to know – although we still feel we let her down.'

'The other thing that made me feel sad is that she is a first-year student in her second term. Aisa has got to stick it out at this university for a few more years. It is a disastrous start for her at college.'

Both the presenting doctor and her partner felt so bad about the patient that they had a session together to try to share their feelings of failure and understand where they had gone wrong.

The presenting doctor made the assumption that this attractive 18-year-old girl could work the system. When she found that the patient had not revealed the whole story and that she chose to go to a clinic ('I don't know what was the attraction of the clinic'), she felt anger at the patient. This was followed by sympathy for her.

Group's feelings

'One of the difficulties with adolescents is that they find it difficult to work the system. If things go wrong it ends up with the GPs crucifying themselves!'

One member of the group said 'I was irritated and then became angry, and am now thinking this poor kid was trying to pluck up the courage. The attacks back this up.'

Themes

- The patient has seen many health professionals but has not built up a rapport or trust with any of them.
- If young people do not come back, should the GP contact them?

- The patient chooses an emergency surgery, and avoids sharing the problems.
- The older adolescent does not reveal the real problem. It is hidden behind a 'ticket' which is easier to present – in this case thrush.
- Whose responsibility is it to expose the problem? Is it that of the patient or the doctor?
- The GP feels many conflicting emotions and especially failure when the outcome is bad for her patient.
- When things go wrong with adolescent patients, doctors tend to blame themselves.
- The doctor is Asian and the practice is very open and tolerant. The doctor felt that the Asian student would feel able to confide in her. However, it is not *easier* for some patients to talk to a doctor of the same sex and ethnic background. In fact it can sometimes be harder.

Overriding emotions

- Presenter: annoyed, angry, frustrated, sad, guilty, 'gutted', 'let her down'.
- Group: empathy, irritation, sadness.

Group leader's comments

This case caused the presenting GP and her practice a great deal of distress. In an attempt to provide easy access, the system inadvertently discouraged continuity and therefore the opportunity for a trusting doctor–patient (or nurse–patient) relationship to develop. There was plenty of 'advice' from various sources, but sadly the opportunity to 'diagnose' the real problem was missed in the frenetic activity. This case illustrates Balint's 'dilution of responsibility'. It may have been that this Asian patient deliberately chose to avoid a deeper relationship, especially with the Asian doctor, for fear of criticism by someone from a similar culture. The doctor's counter-transference is demonstrated by the comment that 'Aisa was not willing to play by adult rules.'

Chapter 10

Case 10: 'Jyoti' – tolerating confusion

Presenter:	GP: female, white.
Patient:	Jyoti: 18 years old, female, Asian.
Setting:	Four visits to the GP at the university practice.

What happened

- *Contact 1: Jyoti visits the GP at the university practice, alone.*
  'She came in looking trendy – tight trousers, leather jacket and a lot of make-up. She wanted emergency contraception, and after discussing this with her I prescribed it. I also told her she could come back and see me if she wanted to.'
- *Contact 2: Jyoti visits the GP at the university practice, alone.*
  She returned for the pill. She had in the past seen an endocrinologist who had prescribed the pill because she was 'very hairy'. Nothing abnormal was found, but she was prescribed the pill. She was coming for a repeat prescription. She said 'Look how hairy I am.' 'I was not convinced.'
  'I suggested she should have a smear, but she didn't want one at that time.'
  Jyoti was due to go home for the holidays. 'We discussed how she felt about this. She told me that her parents had found a man for her, and she was to go to Toronto during the break to meet him. She said she saw this as a way of having a holiday away from the family. She added "I have no intention of marrying him."' The doctor said 'I felt I was being sucked into something. Distrust is too strong a word. She was smiling, but it was a false smile – a façade. I felt she wasn't letting me in. It was all very confusing.'
- *Contact 3: Jyoti visits the GP at the university practice, alone.*
  'She returned three months later for a repeat prescription. I said "Would you like a smear today?" She was a bit reluctant, but said yes. During the examination I touched her vagina and she flinched. I reassured her, explained what I was doing and encouraged her to relax, but she flinched again and said it was painful. It came to my mind that she hadn't ever had sex. So I asked her if it was painful when she had sex. She said "sometimes" but did not sound very convincing.'
  'I asked if she had had full intercourse, and she said "Oh yes", but it did not sound at all convincing. I did not feel I could explore this any more. I thought of referring her for psychosexual counselling, but I didn't. I am not quite sure why.'

- *Contact 4: Jyoti visits the GP at the university practice, alone.*
'I was soon to leave the practice. I broached the subject of psychosexual counselling. I thought it might help her perception of her hairiness as well.

'As she was leaving she turned and said "I just need emergency contraception."'

'I just saw a circle in front of my eyes! I admit at that point I just gave it to her. There wasn't time to say "Do you really need it? Is it to convince yourself that you are sexually active?" I felt I had not moved forward with her. I had this feeling of frustration knowing that there was pretence, in a much divided young person – her choice appeared to be returning to her family culture and a possible arranged marriage or continuing with her Western college life. Her real self was disguised behind her leather jacket and all her make-up. If I was not leaving the practice it would have been a real challenge to get to the bottom of it!'

Doctor's feelings

- 'I didn't warm to her. I just did not feel maternal.'
- 'I thought it was a challenge to resolve what was going on.'
- 'I felt guilty because I was leaving the practice. You get all this information given to you and the patient puts all their trust in you, and you leave.'

Group's feelings

The group found it hard to respond emotionally to the confused patient, as she seemed to be hidden behind a façade.

She did keep coming back to the doctor, which the group thought was positive. However, she kept throwing into the picture new and bizarre things which did not add up. Was she deluded? Was she even psychotic? Or was she unable to decide which cultural attitude to sex and marriage she was going to embrace?

There was a discussion about the fear that Hindu girls often have of seeing 'Hindu doctors', because they are seen as part of the Hindu community and the patient fears they may disclose confidential information.

There was also discussion about how temporary many doctors in practice may be.

Finally, the group discussed GPs' tendency to feel omnipotent and so drive themselves to think they must sort out every problem.

Themes

- The adolescent does not reveal the real problem. She presents a confusing picture.
- The patient chooses to disclose information at the end of a consultation when time is too limited.
- Whose responsibility is it to expose the problem? Is it that of the patient or the doctor?
- Feelings of omnipotence put an impossible load on the doctor.

- GPs cannot resolve young people's difficulties in deciding what culture and sexual attitudes they will adopt.
- It takes time for some adolescents to build up enough confidence in a doctor to enable them to share embarrassing personal conflicts over sexual or cultural attitudes.
- Seeing a patient many times while trust is being built up is not 'doing nothing'.
- It is uncomfortable for a GP to consider psychosis as a possible diagnosis.

Overriding emotions

- Presenter: challenged, distrusting, confused, despairing, guilty, taken aback, 'sucked in', not maternal.
- Group: 'things are not as they seem', support for the GP, surprise, feeling of being taken aback, confusion.

Group leader's comments

The doctor did not warm to this patient, and the group also found it difficult to respond emotionally to her. It was difficult for an effective doctor–patient relationship to develop. The words 'confused' and even 'psychotic' were used, and she was described as being 'hidden behind a façade'. Perhaps it was this lack of openness and the difficulty in believing the patient's story which we found hard. Or was it because we felt that we were being asked to take sides in her disagreement with her family and culture? Was it the lack of an effective doctor–patient relationship which prevented an identification of the 'real diagnosis'?

Chapter 11

Summary of themes emerging from the consultations

In this chapter we classify the themes identified in the discussions (*see* Chapters 1 to 10 in Part 2) under ten headings. We have added to these headings some points that GPs and practice nurses might find it useful to consider when reflecting on their own consultations. Some of the headings address areas that influence the consultation from outside, while others arise from the interaction itself.

1 Building a trusting relationship

This is a central activity in all consultations, but with adolescents it can be particularly difficult. It often takes time – sometimes several contacts. The young patient needs to be seen alone or with a friend and given an environment in which they can get over their embarrassment. To help them, the professional needs to convey that he or she is interested, is prepared to listen and is non-judgemental. Much of this is conveyed by non-verbal communication, including eye contact, tone of voice, posture, facial expression and diplomatic use of notes or computer screen.

The professional also needs to listen carefully to what the adolescent is trying to say, and to read his or her body language with care. These skills are generally poorly taught during training, and it takes practice and awareness to develop them. Until a trusting relationship is established it is unlikely that an adolescent will reveal his or her troubled feelings and personal problems, or listen to any suggestions that are made by the GP or practice nurse.

2 The role of the family

For most adolescents their family provides their greatest source of support. Yet as independence develops there are many areas of their personal life that adolescents wish to keep private.

At the same time, all families have their interpersonal dynamics. In some cases this can include serious complications such as divorce and, rarely, abuse, alcoholism and sometimes debilitating illnesses in other family members. It can then be difficult for the GP or practice nurse to disentangle family from adolescent problems. The fact that the parent may also be a patient of the GP or practice nurse can make the situation even more difficult.

Parents can also hold strong views about how their children should behave – for example, how tidy they should keep their bedrooms, or what religious or cultural behaviour they should follow. Parents sometimes try to use their GP to support these views, and in doing so can exert pressure on the GP to break confidentiality. Parents may also resent the young adolescent seeing the GP on his or her own.

It is important for professionals to respect the role of the family while also respecting the rights and developing independence of their adolescent patients.

3 Diagnosing the 'real' problem

Behind the problem first presented by an adolescent there can be a 'serious condition'. It can take quite a time for some young people to become confident enough to share with a GP or practice nurse that, for example, they are terrified that they could be pregnant, or they feel life is not worth living, or they are taking drugs.

The difficulty for the professional is in deciding how long to wait for confidence to build and how much to probe, remembering all the time that the initial problem may be all that the adolescent is worried about.

4 Whose responsibility?

How far should a professional respect the right of adolescents to make their own decisions? For example, if a young patient with a major problem such as depression does not return to see the GP, should the GP try to contact them? This problem can apply to adolescents with eating disorders or early psychosis, or to patients with a chronic condition such as diabetes who are taking their medication erratically.

Ideally, the professional and patient work together, sharing responsibility. Only if there is a risk of serious harm to themselves or to others does the question of 'chasing up' or sectioning the patient occur (*see also* Appendix 3).

5 Confidentiality

It is essential to reassure adolescents that information given in the consultation is confidential, and that the whole practice supports this ruling. Yet there are situations where confidentiality has to be broken – albeit after informing the patient. The dividing line between normal sexual activity and sexual abuse is a case in point. This raises many difficult issues (for more information on this subject, *see* Appendix 3). For further insight into the issue of confidentiality, the reader is referred to the Confidentiality and Young People toolkit (for details, *see* Part 6).

6 The temptation to slip into a 'parental role'

It is natural for a concerned adult to want to protect an adolescent from harm. However, the professional role is a different one. It is to work *with* our patients – by giving them appropriate information so that they can make their own choices and solve their own problems. This is achieved by respecting their growing autonomy, and by encouraging them to take on responsibility for their own protection, health and welfare, and seeking appropriate help when necessary.

There are times when GPs need to share their views (even if not asked to do so) – for example, on the effects of lack of exercise, anger with teachers and school, unprotected sexual intercourse, or taking drugs and binge drinking. It can be difficult to know how far to go in giving this kind of information without appearing judgemental, and if the balance tips too far in the wrong direction, the consultation can be unproductive.

7 Discussing topics openly

Many professionals as well as many adolescents find it hard to discuss certain topics openly. Examples might include feelings of anger or unhappiness, religious and cultural differences (e.g. arranged marriages), homosexual practices, different forms of drug taking, impending death of a parent or sibling, or possibly sexual abuse or rape (*see* Appendix 3). Discussion can sometimes be more difficult if the GP and the patient are of different gender or ethnic background. It can also be blocked by the use of jargon or religious terms if these are not understood and explained, or if non-verbal signs are misread. For example, lack of eye contact does not necessarily mean lack of attention on the part of the adolescent. Indeed discussion can sometimes be blocked unconsciously by the doctor or practice nurse as a defence mechanism.

Professionals can always share with others the difficulties they are experiencing with their patient and suggest a referral to someone who is more at ease discussing the subject. The important point is to be aware of the topics that one finds difficult and to do something about it.

8 Lack of continuity of care

Most patients would like to continue to see the same GP or practice nurse if they have formed a positive relationship with them. Indeed many GPs feel that, if the patient returns, this is a confirmation that a relationship has been formed. Equally, it is sometimes assumed that the professional 'hasn't got it right' if the patient does not come back.

Yet it is becoming increasingly difficult in some practices for patients to choose whom they can see, and for emergency care they are likely to see a different person. Communication back to the GP then becomes particularly important, but it is not always effective. Also there are many places where adolescents can go for help, such as Brook clinics, genito-urinary medicine (GUM) clinics, Accident and Emergency departments or university practices. The adolescent's GP may never hear from many of these organisations, sometimes because of confidentiality issues. Even referral to specialist care can lead to confusion over who is to be the 'lead physician'.

This lack of continuity of care can make the GP or practice nurse feel upset or anxious, or it may make them think "Why bother?" It could be that patient-held records for this age group might help to overcome this problem of increasing fragmentation of care.

9 Blaming oneself when things go wrong, and other feelings

Things can go terribly wrong with adolescent patients. When a young patient commits suicide, or unintentionally becomes pregnant, or dies with a needle in their arm, the whole practice can feel 'bad'. Often the GP blames him- or herself and may overreact in consultations with other adolescents.

Where do GPs go for support or supervision when this happens? Should practices do more to support each other when difficult feelings arise? All of those who participated in this project agreed that sharing the feelings they had had – sometimes for months – as a result of their 'difficult adolescent consultation' had been very helpful.

Below is a list of all the feelings that were expressed in these discussions. It shows how much GPs do react to these adolescent consultations. Does this age group bring out stronger feelings than other patients? And what harm can these feelings do to the ongoing work of professionals?

Doctors' emotions

'Adolescent'	Impatient
Agitated	Impotent
Angry	Irritated
Annoyed	Manipulated
Anxious	Omnipotent
Challenged	'Parental'
Concerned	Protective
Confused	'Put-upon'
Despairing	Relieved
Distrusting	Sad
Empathic	Surprised
Frustrated	Uncertain
Guilty	Uneasy
Helpless	Unsupported

---

10 Pressure on professionals in primary care

Many professionals in general practice feel under considerable pressure – to maintain quality of care, to keep to time, not to keep other patients waiting, to get out on their 'visits' (i.e. to keep their surgery working effectively and efficiently). There is also pressure from NHS bureaucracy and the fear of litigation and an increasing number of patient complaints.

With adolescents there is often a feeling that 'something must be done' to solve a problem that cannot be solved by a quick medical intervention. This is made more difficult by the current long waiting-time for referrals, especially for psychiatric and drug-related problems.

Many professionals feel under particular pressure to 'get it right' with adolescents, as these young people are on the threshold of adult life, and this could be a last opportunity to steer them in a productive direction – but also because the GP is demonstrating what GP services can offer and conditioning how their patient may use these services in the future.

There is a danger that all of these pressures can undermine a GP's effectiveness. Professionals need to care for themselves as well as for their patients. Those who become over-stressed are of little help to their next patient.

For some it can be helpful to remember that just being present for an adolescent – being concerned and listening, and suggesting a return visit – is in fact 'doing something'. This alone can be therapeutic for the adolescent patient. Realising that not all problems have an immediate solution can also help to take some of the pressure off the professional.

Part 3

Factors that can affect adolescent consultations

The themes that the group identified in the case presentations described in Part 2 point to areas where difficulties are likely to arise in future adolescent consultations. To understand why this is so for this age group, we need to look in more depth at the factors that can influence young patients and the professionals they consult. This section considers the following:

- parents
- the effect of NHS structures
- lack of adequate training
- confusion over where responsibility lies
- the doctor's feelings
- the developmental process among adolescents
- adolescents' views of primary care.

Chapter 1

Parents

Many parents believe that they should accompany their teenage children whenever they visit the GP or practice nurse. One parent said to a member of the group:

What would the doctor think of me if I did not go to the surgery with him?

In a survey of 5152 young people aged 15–16 years, 60% reported that a parent sat in on their last GP consultation.[1] When these contacts are for physical problems, this may not matter. It is when the problem is personal that the presence of the parent can result in communication difficulties. Yet even when the problem is physical, the parent's presence can inhibit the adolescent and GP from discussing important personal areas such as smoking, alcohol consumption, drugs or sexual behaviour. Even if the parent withdraws and enables the young patient to practise consulting on their own and to build their own relationship with their GP, it can lead to concerns. Just knowing that their mother is in the adjacent room and is likely to ask questions on the way home, or knowing that she will want to come to the pharmacist to collect the prescriptions, may be an embarrassment to the adolescent and inhibit openness.

In this project, the group noted that a parent was either present or in the mind of the patient, and often in the mind of the professional, during the majority of the consultations that were discussed. Despite the difficulties this can cause, the parents' attendance illustrates that they provide the main support in many adolescents' lives, and this needs to be respected.

In order to understand the difficulties faced by teenagers, it is worth considering the options that are open to them when they have a problem that they feel they are unable to share with their parents. These are as follows.

- Option 1: do nothing.
- Option 2: provide a 'ticket' explanation.
- Option 3: see the GP alone.

Option 1: do nothing

The hope here is that the problem will go away. Examples of problems where this option might be chosen include being bullied, distress over the break-up of the parents' marriage or relationship, worries over the health of other members of the family, and concern about binge drinking, bulimia or depression. This option is especially attractive to boys with low self-esteem, who believe that they should stand on their own two feet and that seeking help is a sign of weakness.

If the problem does not get better on its own, the behaviour of the teenager may in time become a concern to their family or their school. This behaviour may then be presented at the surgery. If an adult remains at the consultation, the GP may be left totally confused as to how much the presented problem is that of the patient and how much it is that of the adult[1] (*see* Case A).

Option 2: provide a 'ticket' explanation

Another option is for the adolescent to provide his or her family with a 'ticket' explanation. This in turn may be presented at the surgery. Some common 'tickets' are headaches, tiredness or PMT. The GP may then be tempted to treat the ticket problem and, unless he or she is careful, may not hear the real problem at all.

Option 3: see the GP alone

The third option is for the adolescent to access the GP on their own, hoping that their family will not find out. This requires confidence. The teenager needs to get to the surgery without being seen by friends of the family. The receptionist has to be negotiated, friends avoided in the waiting area, and the GP consulted on their own, possibly for the first time. Again a common gambit is to use a 'ticket of entry' in order to provide time to assess the GP.

As the cases presented in Part 2 have shown, even when they have left home, some adolescents find it hard to present their 'real problem' straight away. This can be especially difficult when their family holds strong religious and cultural beliefs. The patient may then assume that the GP will judge them in the same way as their parents. Under this option, 'thrush' may be presented rather than the fear of being pregnant after having unprotected sex, or 'acne' instead of a request for the contraceptive pill.

The parent's view

As children develop through their teens it is very hard for parents to accept that their children are becoming increasingly independent and taking greater responsibility for their own life and health. To keep out of their teenager's problems when they are in difficulty is sometimes asking too much of a caring parent! Yet this is an inevitable part of growing up. Sometimes the process can be made more acceptable if it is discussed with the GP during the early stages of development, at around the age of 12 or 13 years, and if both parent and GP accept that it can be helpful for the teenager to consult on their own and to take increasing responsibility for their health and well-being.

The doctor's view

For the doctor, the whole process of being torn between working with a parent (whom they may have known for many years) and a teenager who is becoming more independent can be difficult. Again the situation can be made easier if it is discussed early on, at the start of puberty. However, the need for confidentiality must be rigorously maintained if adolescents are to have any confidence in using the surgery services in the future. It is not surprising that some adolescent consultations can feel difficult for all concerned!

The role of the family

Adolescents are part of a family group where all kinds of tensions and interpersonal dynamics take place. Loyalty to one's parents, even in families where a youngster is being abused, can be strong. Some teenagers believe that their parents' unhappiness, drinking or separation is in part their responsibility, and that it is their task to support or at least not to contribute to their parents' worries by adding their problem. Serious illness in the family, or bereavement, can also distract attention from a teenager's struggles. Often the problems of the family and the adolescent are so entwined that it takes considerable time in individual or family therapy to disentangle them. Yet GPs are expected to do this in a couple of consultations (*see* Cases A and 2).

Although the 'difficult' consultations highlighted the problems that parents can present, we also need to remember that parents often have a facilitating role in that they are able to convey context and circumstances to a GP more effectively and concisely than an adolescent. However, we cannot over-emphasise the need to see the adolescent alone, if only for part of the consultation, and the need to respect confidentiality.

Many parents find that they agree with this but find it emotionally hard to go along with it when it comes to their own family. At a conference one male GP said: 'I entirely agree with what you are saying, until I think of *my* four daughters. Then I vehemently disagree!'

Reference

1 Donovan C, Mellanby AR, Jacobson LD *et al.* for the RCGP Adolescent Working Party (1997) Teenagers' views on the general practice consultation and provision of contraception. *Br J Gen Pract.* **47**: 715–18.

Chapter 2

The effect of NHS structures

I feel caught by the restraints of the system.
I can't do all that in ten minutes.

(Case 9)

These comments illustrate the influence of the NHS structure within which GPs work.

If these are the responses of those who are interested in adolescent patients, what is likely to be the reaction of those who are not? One hypothesis is that in our surgeries there is much denial of the difficulties that our adolescent patients would like to discuss. One member of the group shared the following with us:

Before I attended the adolescent study day, I too felt that I rarely saw an adolescent patient, but after it I found teenagers of both sexes cluttering up my surgeries.

Perhaps denial, combined with the fact that many adolescent/GP contacts are for relatively simple conditions, has led GPs to use adolescent consultations as a way of catching up on a busy surgery that is running late.

Speculation also led us to think that subconsciously many GPs do not relish probing to find the underlying problems, for fear of opening Pandora's box and finding ourselves landed with a distressing difficult problem which we have neither the time nor the training to handle effectively.

The West Indian boy who was excluded from school in Case 2 is an example of one such problem. It is discouraging to find that the earliest adolescent psychiatric appointment available was in three to six months' time. Social services do not have to accept cases, and drug-dependency units often have long waiting-lists. In short, the fact that training in adolescent medicine for GPs is limited, and back-up secondary care for psychiatry is not well provided for in the NHS, can discourage some primary care professionals from interacting for any length of time with young patients who themselves have difficulty in disclosing their personal problems. Another example was the ignoring of the phrase 'Someone forced me into it [having sexual intercourse]' (see Case 1).

Perhaps this is the result of a service in which the mean consultation time for all patients is said to be 9.4 minutes (in contrast with 10.2 minutes in The Netherlands, 15 minutes in Belgium and 15.6 minutes in Switzerland), and the lack of training in consultation skills for GPs and nursing staff.[1]

The participants did not draw attention to the lack of financial incentives in the present GP contract to encourage quality care for adolescent patients. The new GP contract does not make any significant allowance for fostering longer consultations for this or any age group, except within the broader remit of lengthening overall consultation times. Previous research has demonstrated that teenage consultations are shorter than consultations for other age groups.[2] There will be no overt, specific 'rewards' for longer consultations with teenage patients within the proposed new structure of general practice.

Other problems are also developing within the NHS structure. Referral to specialist care (especially for those with mental health and drugs problems) is taking longer and longer, even for urgent appointments. In some parts of the UK it is even difficult to access GUM clinics.

Continuity of care is becoming a rarity. The new GP contract is not designed to encourage building of relationships with adolescent patients, or to encourage these patients to continue with one professional.

References

1   van den Brink-Muinen A, Verhaak P, Bensing J et al. (2003) Communication in general practice: differences between European countries. *Fam Pract.* **20:** 478–85.
2   Jacobson L, Wilkinson C and Owen P (1994) Is the potential of teenage consultations being missed? A study of consultation times in primary care. *Fam Pract.* **11:** 296–9.

Chapter 3

Lack of adequate training

In the UK, relatively few GPs receive formal training in adolescent health in general, or receive tips on how to consult with teenagers. GPs in the South Wales study (*see also* page xiv earlier) commented that they would value further training in communication skills with this age group.[1] This issue is beginning to receive some attention in other countries, such as Australia and the USA. This study has delineated several communication issues which can add to our understanding of communication when consulting with adolescent patients, and can be regarded as useful background training information for those who will be consulting with teenagers. The issue is also highlighted in a recent report from an Intercollegiate Working Party.[2]

The consultation

Much has been written about what needs to be learnt and taught about the consultation. Silverman, Kurtz and Draper[3] state that:

> Having a structure prevents consultations from wandering aimlessly and important points being missed.

These authors base their structure on five communication skills:

1 initiating the session
2 gathering information
3 building relationships
4 explanation and planning
5 closing the session.

This is appropriate for most adult consultations. However, contact with adolescents – especially those with an embarrassing problem – calls for a slightly different approach.

A different emphasis in consultations with adolescents

All GPs are aware of the need to keep to time. Patients waiting to see them, the desire to keep their appointment system working to time and the need to see their seriously sick patients without too much delay all exert pressure. In an adult consultation, after a welcome by the GP a simple question such as 'What can I do for you today?' will generally produce the patient's account of their problem, and the professional will take a history.

When faced with an adolescent – especially one with an embarrassing personal problem –

a trusting relationship has to be forged first before disclosure is likely to occur. The teenager may well view the GP as an authority figure who may judge them unfavourably once the problem is revealed, and it is important to defuse this impression. Confidentiality rules may need to be stated (*see* Appendix 4). The impression of a doctor who is caring, sensitive and available to work with the young patient needs to be built up.

This all takes time, especially if the young patient's only previous experience of the GP has been as a child, when the GP worked mainly with their parent. The Court report[4] pointed out that the GP needs to change in the eyes of their young patient and become the adolescent's physician rather than the family doctor. It is unrealistic to expect to achieve this in the first few minutes of the consultation with a teenager who is embarrassed by a personal problem such as drug taking, unprotected intercourse or suicidal thoughts. As we have seen, probing to find out the problem is unlikely to be productive until the doctor–patient relationship feels secure. Thus it is often necessary to build up a relationship with an adolescent patient *before* the GP 'gathers information'. It is sometimes hard for GPs to make this change in consultation structure within the time available.

Some members of our group pointed out that their relationship with the adolescent improved over several contacts. Only then did some patients feel able to disclose their problem. This can be frustrating for a GP who is working under pressure. As one GP said:

> Frustration was the biggest thing I felt . . . I wasn't getting any communication and I feel a lot of GP therapy really comes down to how good communication is in a consultation and that was not happening. I felt I was not getting to the bottom of the problem.

Sometimes it can be tempting to move on to the next appointment, where the GP might be more successful.

Howie[5] has shown that, in order to understand the dynamics of any consultation fully, we should look at it in the context of the whole surgery. Then we can see how the dynamics are affected by what has gone on before, how late the GP is running, and the number of patients who are waiting. In this context it is often tempting for the professional to move on without spending time building a relationship, and as a result the patient's problem is not revealed and not addressed.

The group did not overtly raise any issues about the process by which adolescent patients access consultations in primary care. This may be because participants felt that this was not relevant to their discussions, but clearly it is a responsibility for GPs who organise their service. Adolescents have reported in the past and continue to report that two of their concerns about consultations with their GP are the difficulty in getting an appointment in the first place, and receptionists who lack communication skills or who do not respect confidentiality.

References

1   Jacobson L, Richardson G, Parry-Langdon N *et al.* (2001) How do teenagers and primary healthcare providers view each other? An overview of key themes. *Br J Gen Pract.* **51**: 811–16.
2   Royal College of Paediatrics and Child Care (2003) *Bridging the Gap: health care for adolescents.* Royal College of Paediatrics and Child Care, London.

3 Silverman J, Kurtz S and Draper J (1998) *Skills for Communicating with Patients*. Radcliffe Medical Press, Oxford.

4 Court SDM (1976) *Fit for the Future*. HMSO, London.

5 Howie J (1999) *Patient Centredness and Politics of Change*. John Fry Fellowship, The Nuffield Trust, London.

Chapter 4

Confusion over where responsibility lies

There was a feeling among some in the project group that, despite what has been said, it is the GP's job to read between the lines, interpret non-verbal behaviour and somehow understand the adolescent's underlying problem in the limited time available. If they do not and things go wrong, the GP often blames him- or herself:

> I let her down. I handled it very badly.
>
> (Case 9)

Others pointed out that this is sometimes not possible, and that it is the patient's responsibility to disclose:

> I told her that if she did not tell me what was wrong I could not help her.
>
> (Case A)

The group supported the notion that it is the GP's responsibility to build up an environment of trust while attempting to interpret the signals as best they can, but that they also have a responsibility to see other patients who are waiting. Many of the GPs were concerned about whether the patient would return, as to them this was a sign that they had begun to form a positive relationship. Indeed coming back seemed to be a sign that the GP had 'got it right'. If the patient does not come back, the GP can be left wondering.

> If they disappear, you are left with the feeling you don't know.
>
> (Case 7)

The group felt that there was more worrying about 'getting it right' in adolescent consultations than in adult consultations because if a patient of this age can build a good relationship with a GP, it may set them on a path of using GP services in the future. One member expressed it as follows:

> If she goes away to college she may hope to meet another 'you' there.
>
> (Case 7)

The opposite was also felt:

> The part I feel worse about is not that she is pregnant, but the loss of trust.
>
> (Case 9)

Sometimes a GP may feel guilty about ending a trusting relationship that they have developed with a patient:

> I felt guilty because I left the practice. They invest their trust in you and then you leave.
>
> (Case 10)

There was some confusion about how much GPs should feel responsible for adolescent patients, and how much they should respect the adolescent's ability to handle their own problem (i.e. respect the young patient's growing autonomy).

In one case the GP said:

> I'm worrying about her a lot, but maybe she wasn't asking me to help her with these problems. Maybe it is more my anxiety about the problem.
>
> (Case 7)

The psychiatrist in the group showed us how she demonstrated her trust in her patient who had attempted suicide by agreeing not to pass her on to a colleague when she (the psychiatrist) moved on and felt that her patient was then out of danger (*see* Case 5). This kind of trust can leave the doctor worrying 'Will things go wrong? Will the patient kill herself?' Even criticism from young patients can lead GPs to accept blame.

> She told you – you got it wrong.
>
> (Case 9)
>
> It will be a disaster if you do not get it right.
>
> (Case 4)

Seeing other health professionals can also be interpreted by the first doctor contacted as a sign that 'you did not get it right'. In Case 9 the patient saw an 'on-call' doctor twice, her family GP and a family planning doctor without returning to the original university practice, and the university practice doctor blamed herself.

This raises the question of responsibility. Just as parents transfer trust and responsibility to their teenagers by degrees, so it seems reasonable for GPs to make assumptions about the degree of responsibility a college student can carry as opposed to, say, a 14- or 15-year-old. The more mature the adolescent appears to be, the more the doctor might assume that they have developed the ability to disclose their underlying problem increasingly easily. This assumption can sometimes lead the GP astray.

Chapter 5

The doctor's feelings

Strong feelings were aroused in the GP in most of the consultations discussed. Indeed, it was largely because the GPs were still carrying these feelings that they were prompted to bring the consultation to the group.

Many of the professionals in the group agreed that it was helpful to monitor their feelings during the interaction and to ask 'Is this coming from my patient or from myself?' It was also accepted that discussing their emotions in the group and discovering that colleagues had experienced similar feelings was supportive. Some feelings came up more than others, particularly frustration, anxiety, anger and a sense of failure. These have all been touched upon (*see* page 44). Here we would like to mention four more:

- omnipotence
- impotence
- adolescent or parental feelings
- positive feelings because an interaction has gone well.

Omnipotence

The feeling of omnipotence was acknowledged in the group.

I felt it must be up to the GP to sort it out.

(Case 2)

The group discussed whether it was a weakness for a GP to take on cases that other services had refused or discharged as being beyond help. It was agreed that the GP's role was to recognise distress and be alongside the young patient in that distress, but there was a need to have limits to what can be done by a GP.

This was particularly difficult when the GP felt that it was 'a young life on the brink of disaster'. In these cases, just being there did not feel as if it was enough. 'I didn't know what else to offer except to say we are here.' However, the group felt that being there for the patient, actively listening, and being concerned and ready to see them again was in itself therapeutic, and was often sufficient.

Despite this, the group acknowledged an overriding emotion:

I must get it right or a whole life will be ruined.

(Case 4)

GPs have no built-in supervision of their work. It may be that some GPs' reactions were stimulated by their experiences with regard to their own unresolved adolescent problems, and that some kind of supervision or Balint work would benefit them. Certainly being aware of our limitations is no bad thing, especially if we seek further training to modify them.

Impotence

Some GPs felt that the challenge was too much, and this led them into confusion and help-lessness:

> I felt I was being sucked into something.
>
> (Case 10)

> The feeling I had was that of going around in a circle. I just saw a circle in front of my eyes.
>
> (Case 10)

> I just felt a bit impotent and did not know what I could do.
>
> (Case A)

In some of the presentations, the group felt that the doctor's confusion reflected the adolescent's confusion. In others, the problem was just too complicated.

> I feel she is very vulnerable, but don't know how to help her.
>
> (Case 7)

> I felt I had not moved forward maybe half an inch and felt quite depressed.
>
> (Case A)

Yet others argued that being available, forming a relationship and letting the young patient see that the GP is concerned is 'doing something', however hard it feels for the GP who wishes to solve all of the problems that their adolescent patient is carrying. It comes down to a matter of attitude – just listening and showing concern for the young person's problem is 'doing something'.

The doctor who is experiencing parental or adolescent feelings

Knowing the whole family, and seeing the children grow up, can make it difficult for a doctor not to identify with the parent. In short it is hard for GPs not to experience parental feelings – to be protective, and to fight the adolescent's problems for them rather than respecting their autonomy and their right to 'get it wrong'.

GPs can also have the experience of slipping into reacting like an 'adolescent' themselves. In one case the GP said:

I could hear myself in adolescent mode.

(Case 4)

This can happen when a teenager questions the GP's authority, or when they say 'You got it wrong.' Being aware that many GPs can be upset in this way, and also being aware of it at the time of the consultation, can be both helpful and – as we have seen – productive.

Positive emotions

This project has looked at the feelings generated in difficult consultations with adolescents. Although the group agreed that it can be hard to win the confidence of adolescents and open up the channels of genuine communication, this is not always the case. Members agreed that there were many consultations in which adolescents had proved to be fantastic patients (*see* page 95, on What do young people tell ChildLine about their doctors?). Once they trust the GP, adolescents can be more open and honest and less inhibited than adults, and make full use of their professional contacts.

The group agreed that consultations with adolescent patients can be one of the more satisfying aspects of general practice, and that the implications of the group's discussions may be unrepresentative of all the consultations taking place with teenage patients. The group indicated that their discussions had necessarily been based on difficult consultations, and an exploration of why they were perceived to have been difficult, but that this was not the full story.

At the end of the group meetings, participants indicated that a further project involving exploration of 'successful adolescent consultations', the emotions these aroused and the perceptions of why they had been successful was also worthy of study. This aspect of doctors' training and culture, where self-criticism is regarded as more worthy of reportage than any form of self-praise, has implications beyond this work, but warrants future exploration.

Chapter 6

The developmental process in adolescents

Adolescents vary as much as patients in other age groups. For some adolescents a consultation can be a daunting and embarrassing process, while for others – perhaps those who have received much medical care on account of a chronic health problem such as diabetes or cancer – it can be almost commonplace.

Yet even those who are used to consultations can, when they pass through puberty, find that revealing intimate details about themselves is so embarrassing that they cannot face it, and as a result they may block discussing their 'real problem'.

The changes that take place around puberty are well known. We mention a few of these changes below, as a reminder of the profound influence that they can have on adolescent patients.

Physical changes

Dramatic changes in the bodies of teenagers can cause a variety of feelings. Some teenagers are proud of these, while others are horrified or ashamed. Almost all are anxious to seek reassurance that what is happening to them is normal.

These worries are often heightened by a lack of information about the changes before they occur, and by the fact that changes occur at different times for different individuals. Those who mature early or late in particular can feel out of step with their average classmates. Many of these anxieties are kept from adults. Concerns about penis size and masturbation may cause as much anxiety for boys as periods or breast development do for girls.

The establishment of a trusting relationship is essential before a young person is likely to consider sharing their worries with an adult relative, let alone with a professional. Even then, it is often easier to confide in an adult of the same sex. In short, it is unrealistic to expect a young adolescent to visit a GP whom they hardly know, and to quickly reveal their intimate feelings to them.

Emotional changes

The eruption of powerful feelings and violent mood swings is characteristic of the teenage years. Much of this takes place in a private world and may be shared only with peers or a diary. Parents tend to see only changes in behaviour and emotional outbursts, which demonstrate the tip of a developing emotional iceberg.

Teenagers may not understand these waves of emotion themselves. A young girl may just sit and weep and not know why (*see* Case A on page 6). A young man, to his distress, may act out his anger, hit his teacher and be unable to explain why (*see* Case 2 on page 15). It is this altered behaviour that can be presented at the surgery by parents (it is worth mentioning that half of the adolescent problems discussed by the group were in fact presented by adults).

Part of this emotional world will contain strong sexual impulses, which can lead adults to develop real and imaginary fears. Teenagers can feel guilt about these feelings. Some seriously dislike the person they are becoming, and attack themselves or lapse into depression rather than share their feelings with an adult. Others may block their feelings with drink, drugs or anti-social behaviour rather than seek help.

Disclosure in the consultation may be very hard, and inevitably it takes time. Some adolescents who get as far as the GP's room may start the consultation by playing for time. Many produce a simple physical problem such as spots or PMT as a 'ticket of entry'. This gives the young patient time to assess the mood of the professional and to see whether they can relate to them.

As we have already seen, the professional can at this point all too easily send out signals that will ensure a short consultation. However, if there is a wish to uncover the patient's 'real problem', the professional might deal sympathetically but quickly with the 'ticket', and then concentrate on building a non-threatening relationship. This can be done by asking general questions about schoolwork or interests, rather than probing into personal activities such as smoking or sexual practices, which would hint at professional judgements.

This is not to say that gentle probing is not sometimes helpful – but that being friendly and giving the patient space and time has a place in enabling them to gain the confidence necessary to share their inner world. This may take more than one or two contacts, and many professionals are not able to provide this.

Cognitive abilities

The ability to explore and formulate hypotheses develops slowly during mid-adolescence. This development enables a teenager to make 'higher-order constructs' and leads to them forming their own 'values' and 'ideals'.

Inevitably, this leads to questioning of the values held by parents and other adults. To begin with this is done in secret, but in time confrontations may take place. This can occur in relatively safe areas such as how tidy to keep one's bedroom (*see* Case 3). In time, however, some adolescents may develop the conviction that they hold superior values to those of adults.

Adolescent criticism of adult 'values' can be projected on to GPs, making it hard for the adolescent to confide in someone whom they believe is practising by inadequate standards of care, concern or confidentiality.

Difficulty in revealing the 'real problem'

Adolescents show great variation when consulting. For some, inexperience in making consultations on their own, combined with the newness and fragility of their inner emotional world and a fear of being judged by adults, can make it difficult for them to seek help and, even if they do, to reveal personal problems to a professional whom they hardly know.

If this situation is not to lead to difficulty, it requires a sensitive response by the professional – for example, carefully reading the young person's body language, providing time in which a relationship of trust can be established, and concerned listening – so that confidence is built up, a relationship of trust develops and the real problem is eventually shared.

As we shall see on page 70, these are resources that GPs practising in the busy NHS often find it difficult to provide.

Chapter 7

Adolescents' views of primary care

When adolescents think of consulting their GP, their views about local primary care services may condition how they behave. For professionals who are aiming to help them, it is important to be aware of these views and to take them into account both when organising their surgery and in the consultation. This chapter provides a brief summary of some of what we know about adolescent views of primary care gathered from five recent research projects.

A project in North London

In a research project conducted in North London schools, 347 young people aged 12–18 years completed a questionnaire in class.[1] This indicated the difficulties that they experienced when consulting a GP. The most common difficulty was embarrassment about discussing personal concerns, experienced by 45% of males and 65% of females. Almost 50% of teenagers (both male and female) had difficulty in obtaining a quick appointment. About 20% of males and 32% of females found their doctor unsympathetic, and a similar proportion of males and females were concerned that their parents would find out about the consultation.

The Northumberland Project

Between 1996 and 1998, the Northumberland Project ran sessions for young people away from NHS surgeries and collected teenage views on the medical profession.[2] The most important characteristics they would like to see in professionals working in primary care are listed in Table 1.

Table 1 Young people's views on the most important characteristics of professionals working in primary care*

Being able to respect confidentiality	83%
Being able to listen	81%
Not being shocked and judging me	74%
Having an idea of what it is like to be a young person now	62%
Not jumping down your throat and saying 'Don't do that'	59%
Helping me to make my own decisions	50%
Not acting as if he or she knows best	44%

*Items are listed in order of the number of young people classifying the item as very important. $n = 707$.
Source: McNulty and Turner.[2]

The South Wales Project

The South Wales Project provided information from 1082 questionnaires completed by 14- to 18-year-olds (with a 49% response rate) and the views of 31 teenagers interviewed in groups.[3]
  The researchers reported the following findings.

- Adolescents have a lack of knowledge of the services available from primary care.
- Adolescents believe that professionals lack respect for teenagers' health concerns.
- Adolescents claim that GPs have poor communication skills.
- There is poor understanding of confidentiality.

Consultation times

In total, 21% of adolescents complained that their time with the doctor was not long enough. The consultation length was under 5 minutes for about a third of the teenagers (33%), and fewer than 10 minutes for 50% of them.

Attitude of GPs

The researchers wrote:

> The focus groups appear to value those doctors who allowed them time to overcome their initial fears and gain confidence to voice their concerns. These characteristics enabled them to relax, and came from GPs who are caring, friendly, interested and who listen.

Adolescents who do not feel relaxed when consulting claim that this is associated with GPs who are:

> patronising, judgemental and superior and who do not listen.

One teenager said:

> I'm really intimidated when I go to my doctor. I sit there and say 'Yes doctor' and 'No doctor'.

Confidentiality

The fear that some of the information divulged in the consultation would be fed back to their family was an ongoing concern for many adolescents:

> Teenagers know that the service is confidential, but individually they worry their doctor will tell their parents.

The authors claimed that there were still some younger patients (i.e. under 16 years of age) who reported that their surgery had a policy that patients under 16 years had to be accompanied by an older relative.

In the commentary, the authors wrote:

> Many teenagers reported apprehension about making an appointment with primary care professionals. They expressed a reluctance to approach receptionist staff, a lack of respect from the surgery team, and a perception of being stereotyped.

Poor communication skills

An important view reported by the authors was that communication skills among doctors were poor. Other studies have made the point that many teenagers feel uncomfortable in their GP's surgery.[4] The South Wales Project confirms this view. One teenager said:

> It's not that he doesn't listen. Sometimes he doesn't fully comprehend that he is talking in a way you can't understand.

A survey of teenagers in Barking and Havering

In this project, 1045 adolescents completed a questionnaire in Barking and Havering district.[5] Although 75% of them were positive about being given helpful advice at a consultation, 54% (567 individuals) thought that they had to be over 16 years of age to access sexual health services, and 58% (604 individuals) were concerned that confidentiality would not be preserved. Concerns that GPs did not have the time or the skills to deal with their problem were expressed by 30%, and a third of the sample felt that GPs would not understand their problem.

Teenagers showed a strong preference for seeing a GP of the same sex. More males (68%) than females (39%) preferred to see the GP on their own. The lower percentage of girls who preferred to see the GP on their own was partly accounted for by the fact that some girls preferred to see the GP with a friend. In this study only 13% of adolescents (more girls than boys) would choose to see a GP with a parent.

In the discussion section the author questions why so few adolescents see the GP without a parent if their preference is to consult on their own. The author asks whether parents insist on attending, or refuse to let the adolescent consult alone, or whether teenagers are unable to tell their parents their preference. Alternatively, it is asked, are many GPs unaware of adolescents' rights? The author concludes that:

> whatever the reasons, the wishes and views of the individual, teenagers do not appear to be understood or realised by parents or practitioners.

The findings of this research should encourage GPs and practice nurses to suggest that the last part of a parent-attended consultation should be held with the patient alone.

A survey of five practices in the East Midlands

In a study by Churchill *et al.*,[6] postal questionnaires were sent to teenagers aged 13–15 years in five practices in the East Midlands. These were analysed to distinguish between those who had 'potential attitudinal barriers' to general practice and those who did not. These were then compared with actual consultation data from retrospective case-note analysis for the preceding 12 months. Matched data were available for 678 adolescents. The project found some overall differences in the use of GPs.

Differences did exist in their perceived difficulties in getting an appointment, their feeling able to confide in the GP, and their perception of adequate time being given in the consultation. The authors state:

> Embarrassment was a more widely expressed concern, especially amongst girls, and such concerns were shown to be associated with reduced consultation for sensitive problems such as gynaecological and contraceptive reasons.

The authors conclude:

> Previously reported negative attitudes of teenagers towards general practice appear to have a limited inhibitory effect on their use of services. However, our study confirms the need for GPs to try to develop trusting relationships with their teenage patients so that they are more likely to confide, and be less embarrassed to do so when they have health concerns.

References

1 Kari J, Donovan C, Li J and Taylor B (1997) Adolescents' attitudes to general practice in North London. *Br J Gen Pract.* **47**: 631–4.
2 McNulty A and Turner G (1998) *Not Just a Phase We're Going Through. Final Report of Northumberland Young People's Health Project 1996–1998*. Child Health Clinic, Ashington.
3 Jacobson L, Richardson G, Parry-Langdon N *et al.* (2001) How do teenagers and primary healthcare providers view each other? An overview of key themes. *Br J Gen Pract.* **51**: 811–16.
4 Donovan C, Mellanby AR, Jacobson LD *et al.* for the RCGP Adolescent Working Party (1997) Teenagers' views on the general practice consultation and provision of contraception. *Br J Gen Pract.* **47**: 715–18.
5 Burack R (2000) Teenagers' attitudes towards general practitioners and their provision of sexual health care. *Br J Gen Pract.* **50**: 550–54.
6 Churchill R, Allen J, Denman S *et al.* (2000) Do the attitudes and beliefs of young teenagers towards general practice influence actual consultation behaviour? *Br J Gen Pract.* **50**: 953–7.

Part 4

Professionals' perspectives

Chapter 1

A GP's experience

Heather C Suckling

I recall an incident when I was casually asking a patient of 20 years' standing how her three teenage children were. She replied 'Large and loud!' This struck me as an accurate description of many adolescents, and perhaps these factors influence our behaviour towards them.

Until I began to take a particular interest in these consultations I *thought* that I did not see many adolescents, but when I kept a record I found that patients from this age group did consult me, and in considerable numbers. Why had I thought otherwise? What is it about these consultations which failed to remain in my mind?

What are the facts?

- *Consultations with adolescents account for 13% of all consultations in primary care.*
  In a study of a general practice in Cardiff, South Wales, Jacobson *et al.* revealed that of the 900 consultations with the six doctors over a three-month period, 119 consultations were with patients aged 11–19 years.[1]
  Another study[2] reported that 50% of adolescents had visited their GP within the previous six months.
- *A consultation with an adolescent is on average two minutes shorter than other consultations.*
  In the South Wales study[1] the length of all consultations was recorded, and those with patients in the 11–19 years age group were found to be significantly shorter (mean duration 6.38 minutes as opposed to 8.28 minutes).

What were the adolescents consulting me about?

Some adolescents came to the surgery with what could be perceived as minor problems, such as a sprained ankle, an upper respiratory infection, acne, or concern about minor lumps and bumps, or for travel advice or certificates. Others had more serious medical problems when I fear I was less aware of the patient as an adolescent with specific needs. For example, when presented with asthma, diabetes and other chronic conditions, I tended to revert to 'protocol mode'. A third group openly expressed their anxieties about matters such as sexual health, contraceptive problems, pregnancy (real or feared), depression and eating disorders.

I suspect that on many occasions, although I had listened and perhaps advised or treated,

I had failed to find out the real reason why the adolescent had come. I had made assumptions, but how often were these accurate? Had they come to 'test me out', to see if they could trust me with their real problem? Had they hoped to air their fears or express their feelings, but been afraid to do so? Had they feared that I would not respect their confidence or even that I would laugh at them? Had they dropped hints, hoping that I would take them up, only to leave without having the chance to open up?

What were *my* problems?

Once I began to think about these consultations, I came to some uncomfortable conclusions about myself. Unlike consultations with my adult patients, in which I enjoyed the challenge of diagnosis and negotiation with the patient, with adolescents I often felt uneasy. I have tried to analyse some of the reasons for this.

1 I tended to make assumptions about adolescents and what they wanted from me.
2 My behaviour tended to be different, and more defensive, in these consultations.
3 I was conscious of my responsibility to the parents (who may also be my patients). Although the doctor's primary responsibility is to the individual patient, the boundaries are not always clear. There may be a real or perceived conflict of interest. For example, in certain exceptional circumstances the adolescent's right to confidentiality may have to be relinquished, and the doctor and parents may have different views on whether those circumstances apply in their case.
4 I was busy promoting *my* agenda – for example, health promotion issues.
5 I was acutely aware of the lack of adequate resources for adolescents, particularly for secondary-care referrals.
6 I was afraid that I would not be able to cope with the problems presented to me, and that if I delved too deeply I would be overwhelmed. I was afraid of opening Pandora's box.

In 1998 I attended the conference organised by the Adolescent Task Group of the Royal College of General Practitioners, which inspired this book, and it opened my eyes to the fact that I was not alone. Many of my colleagues in primary care, from all disciplines, shared the same difficulties in the consultation. Therefore I was very pleased to have the opportunity to lead a Balint group to try to explore these issues as a pilot research project.

What did I learn from the group?

The work of the group is described in some detail elsewhere in this book, but I shall summarise some of the discoveries which I made as a member of that group.

Problems for the doctor

1 Doctors make the following assumptions about adolescents

- *Adolescents are poor communicators.*
  This is a common assumption, but is it true? It is often the case that adolescents are

somewhat inarticulate and that they use language which is very different from that of adults, but this does not mean that their verbal communication is unclear or ineffective. They tend to be very honest (sometimes brutally so), and this can be disconcerting to the doctor. I realised that sometimes it was convenient for me to say they are inarticulate as a defence against hearing some uncomfortable messages. Adolescents also use body language and behaviour very effectively. Most parents (and health professionals) are only too familiar with glowering or sulky expressions, slammed doors and other aspects of behaviour that an adult would hesitate to exhibit.

- *Adolescents are impatient and intolerant.*
  It is true that adolescents are often reluctant to wait for an appointment, and they give short shrift if they feel that they are being 'palmed off', but in my experience they are genuinely appreciative when their concerns are taken seriously by the health professional or receptionist.
- *There is a hidden agenda.*
  Is there? There may well be, but not always. Some adolescents may use a 'ticket of entry' to start the consultation. For example, a patient may present with a sore throat, testing the GP to see whether the doctor is 'someone you can talk to', but he may equally well have a very sore throat and want to know whether he should be prescribed penicillin. A young person asking for the pill may fear that she is already pregnant, but she may be making a straightforward and responsible request for contraception.
- *I have to get this right.*
  Consultations with adolescents sometimes exaggerate the tendency of the doctor to feel omnipotent. I frequently felt that if a consultation with an adolescent went badly, that would adversely affect the young person for ever. In fact, although it is true that a good consultation can do much to ease future consultations with health professionals, a single negative experience is unlikely to do irreparable damage.
- *All consultations are really about sex.*
  Clearly they are not all about sex. Certainly it is true that sex is particularly important to adolescents. Their feelings and sexual desires can be intense, and they are prone to many anxieties which are related to sex, but it is not helpful to *assume* that this is the real reason for every consultation.
- *She wants the pill.*
  It is important to consider the desire or need for contraception, but it cannot be assumed that it is the pill the young woman wants. If the doctor is a good listener and allows the patient time, she will usually be able to express her real needs. If a young woman is not sexually active, she may be upset by the assumption that she wants the pill. Or she may feel that feel that she *should* be sexually active and that she is in some way abnormal if she is not.
- *The patient is trying to get out of something.*
  Young people may need to consult us in order to obtain a letter or certificate to excuse them from certain activities, such as sports or examinations, but this may not be the only reason for the consultation.

2 Defensive behaviour in the doctor

Doctors need defences to maintain their own emotional health and allow them to function professionally. However, it is important that doctors recognise when they are using them and ensure that they do not interfere with the consultation process. The type of defences will depend on the individual doctor, but those listed below are common, and I find myself using them. Tom Main refers to the need for 'elastic bespoke medical defences tailored for each case and each doctor' rather than 'automatic blind defensive procedures and behaviours', but he also warns against creating general rules.[3]

The following are some commonly used defences.

- *I haven't got enough time.*
  As doctors we frequently use our most well-known and arguably most useful defence 'I haven't got time' or 'A consultation is only 10 minutes. That's not long enough to deal with difficult problems.' However, research shows that in fact we spend *less* time in consultations with adolescents than with other patients. Why is this? It may be that many of the consultations are indeed for simple conditions, but it may equally be that because consultations with adolescents tend to be uncomfortable and worrying, that unconsciously we use the time factor as a defence.
- *How can I help a patient who won't speak to me?*
  The common assumption that adolescents are poor communicators has already been discussed. If the doctor is able to demonstrate respect for the patient and is prepared to listen attentively, this problem can usually be overcome.
- *The patient sees me as an 'old fogy.'*
  The doctor wants to be seen as non-judgemental, to be able to understand the adolescent's language and not to be 'stuffy'. Adopting the attitude that 'they would not want to confide in an old fogy like me' may be a defence against hearing a difficult or distressing problem.
- *I don't want to be intrusive.*
  This is a real fear – a wish to avoid an intrusion into the adolescent's private world, as their need for privacy may border on the paranoid. However, this respect for their privacy, like lack of time, may also be a defence mechanism.
- *I should give health promotion advice.*
  This is an important role for health professionals, but can also be used as a defence against hearing the patient's concerns.

The above are just some examples of defences that doctors commonly use, sometimes inappropriately. To quote from Salinsky and Sackin:[4]

> Some defences are essential if the doctor is to survive and continue to function professionally, but excessive and unnecessary defences simply prevent him from listening with empathy.

3 The relationship between the doctor and the parents of the adolescent

In the presentations by the doctors in the Balint research group (*see* Part 2), it was striking that, even when a parent was not physically in the consulting room, the parent (usually the mother) was very much in the doctor's mind. Possible reasons for this include the following.

- Consultations with adolescents often involve some aspect of the relationship between the adolescent and his or her parents.

- The doctor may have adolescent children (or children who have been through adolescence) of his or her own and identify with the parental role.
- The doctor may have known the patient since early childhood and again identify with the parental role.
- The adolescent may treat the doctor as a surrogate parent or behave in a childlike manner.
- The parents of the adolescent may also be patients of the doctor.

In the Court report[5] it was suggested that the adolescent should have the opportunity to renegotiate their relationship with their GP, so that they could see their doctor as their own physician, rather than as the family doctor. This was emphasised by Donovan *et al.* in their paper on setting up a teenage clinic.[6] They suggested that the adolescent could re-register with another partner or practice. This would help both doctor and patient to see each other in a new light and relate more easily on an adult-to-adult basis.

4 The doctor's agenda

In the present environment, where targets are integral to everyday practice, the doctor has his own or her own agenda for the consultation. This applies particularly to adolescents because of the concern about teenage pregnancy rates, smoking, and alcohol and drug abuse in this age group. This means that there is a temptation to use the consultation to promote preventive measures and a healthier lifestyle, even if this is at the expense of the patient's own concerns. Such unsolicited advice is usually ineffective, and inhibits the full exploration of the *patient's* agenda.

5 Inadequate resources

Identifying psychological problems in adolescents is just the beginning of the process. It is necessary to examine the problem in the context of the patient's family, school or college and the numerous social influences on him or her. This requires a multidisciplinary approach and, although the primary healthcare team is often very effective, when specialist help is needed this is very scarce and the referral process is slow and tortuous. This is demonstrated in Case 2 (*see* page 15), here Harold was excluded from school but had to wait several months before specialist help was available.

6 Pandora's box

Doctors are human, too, and seeing patients can be very stressful. The patient's problems may awaken hidden anxieties and fears in the doctor which relate to his or her own history and experience, both professional and personal. These may surface during the consultation or after the patient has left, with the doctor wishing that the consultation had taken a different course. In his seminal work, *The Inner Consultation*, Neighbour describes the 'housekeeping' component of the consultation.[7] By this he means that after each consultation the doctor should consciously pause to check out his or her own feelings and try to resolve them before the next consultation. This is an effective way of reducing and preventing stress, and the experienced doctor learns to work within his or her limits. It is not possible to examine every one of, say, 40 consultations in a day in depth, so the doctor has to choose which he feels able to cope with on a particular day. It is likely that some consultations with adolescents will not be explored because of the real or perceived risk of uncovering complex, anxiety-provoking, emotionally draining or time-consuming issues.

The above problems all have an effect on the consultation process – they divert the doctor's attention from the patient. The most important quality in a doctor is probably the ability to listen attentively and give the patient undivided attention.[8] This is the essence of Balint's idea of the doctor being the drug – that the experience of the consultation itself is crucial to the therapeutic process.[9] This can be difficult when the doctor is anxious, has a list of hypotheses about the patient's reason for the consultation, is worrying about the patient's parents, and has an agenda of his or her own (such as health promotion), all to be fitted into the consultation. However, there is no doubt that attentive listening is what the patient wants and probably needs.

Problems for the patient

The previous section lists the doctor's problems and how the group helped me to understand them better, but communication is by definition dependent on both parties, so I am going to list some of the patients' problems in the consultation. These are taken from my own experience and the group discussions, but the first five problems are also supported by the findings of Jacobson et al.[10]

- *The doctor will not have time to see me.*
  Adolescents are aware that GPs are busy. They may well have tried to make an earlier appointment, or experienced a hurried consultation. They may also feel that their problems may not be considered important enough to warrant taking up the doctor's time.
- *The doctor will not listen to me.*
  Adolescents, like other patients, need to feel that what they say is being heard and that the doctor is giving them his or her undivided attention. I know from my own experience that this is sometimes difficult, and that my head is full of the messages which I want to convey rather than being free to listen attentively.
- *The doctor won't understand.*
  The cliché 'You don't understand,' which is so often heard from the lips of adolescents, needs to be taken seriously. Perhaps more than anything else the adolescent wants and needs to be understood. This applies the other way round, too: 'It's not that he doesn't listen ... sometimes he doesn't fully comprehend that he's talking in a way you can't understand ... it would help if they talked to teenagers.'[10]
- *The doctor or receptionist may tell my parents/teacher/practice staff/other people who know my family.*
  Confidentiality is a real concern of adolescents, and it is important to make clear the principles of the confidentiality policy. For example, the following should be explained.
  - Doctors, nurses and all health professionals have a duty of confidentiality to patients of all ages, including those under 16 years of age.
  - Confidentiality may only be broken in exceptional circumstances – that is, when the health, safety or welfare of the patient or others would otherwise be at grave risk.
  - Whenever possible, the patient should be informed *before* confidentiality is broken, unless to do so would be dangerous to the patient or others.

It is very helpful if the practice provides written information in the form of posters and leaflets, so that all patients, including the parents of the adolescents, are aware of the rules.[11]

- *The doctor will nag me about smoking/alcohol/drugs/eating/sex.*
  This is probably true! Personally, I have to bite my lip because I do realise that unsolicited advice of this nature is at best ignored and at worst counter-productive.
- *The doctor will think I am stupid and laugh at me.*
  This reflects the lack of confidence and self-esteem of some adolescents, but the fear of being laughed at or thought 'stupid' is a real one. (I recall a particular consultation when a 14-year-old came with a pain in his groin. When I examined him, he was acutely embarrassed and then asked me if I thought the size of his penis was normal. When I was able to reassure him, his relief was clearly evident. I was touched when he thanked me for not laughing at him.)
- *The doctor will psychoanalyse me/think I am mad.*
  It is easy for us, as doctors, to forget that sometimes we are seen as having almost magical powers which enable us to interpret and draw significant and sometimes frightening conclusions from the simplest of conversations. Many adolescents are already anxious that they may not be 'normal', and thus their fear of madness is increased.

Conclusion

The above difficulties are frequently encountered and provide challenges for the doctor. The ability to share experiences and feelings with colleagues in a safe environment was, for me, inestimable. The group experience enabled me to reflect on this aspect of my work as I had never done before, and to realise that I was not alone in finding many consultations with adolescents difficult. It helped me to understand some of the reasons for this, and encouraged me to try to explore my discomfort in the consultation rather than merely suppress it. My defences were still strong, but I was more conscious of them and therefore they were less inhibitory to the doctor–patient relationship.

I would like to think that my subsequent consultations with adolescents were more satisfactory for them, but at least they were less anxiety-provoking for me. Some of the lessons I have learned are summarised briefly below.

- Adolescents deserve at least as much time as my other patients.
- Adolescents are *individuals* who need to be encouraged to take responsibility for their own health, (even if I have known them and their families since early childhood). This may require a renegotiation of my relationship with them.
- Like all my patients they should be treated with respect, even if their behaviour makes this difficult.
- Adolescents really appreciate someone who listens to them attentively, takes their concerns seriously and genuinely tries to understand them.
- Adolescents are forgiving, so even if the health professional does not succeed in helping them to resolve their problems, they give us credit for trying!
- Confidentiality is of the utmost importance to adolescents. What is meant by confidentiality needs to be made explicit, and any exceptions must be discussed with them fully.
- Although lifestyle advice is important it should not take precedence over the patient's

own concerns. Given sensitively and at an appropriate time, it is appreciated by the patient.

- However much the doctor tries to equalise the relationship, it is likely that he or she will be perceived (at least initially) as an authoritarian figure or may be expected to react as a parent.

The value of effective consultations with adolescent patients is incalculable – although it is frequently underestimated by the doctor. Patients, on the other hand, appreciate being listened to, respected and valued as individuals and recognise that a good consultation is helpful to them, whatever their problem.

References

1 Jacobson L, Wilkinson C and Owen P (1994) Is the potential of teenage consultations being missed? A study of consultation times in primary care. *Fam Pract.* **11**: 296–9.

2 Donovan C, Mellanby AR, Jacobson LD *et al.* for the RCGP Adolescent Working Party (1997) Teenagers' views on the general practice consultation and provision of contraception. *Br J Gen Pract.* **47**: 715–18.

3 Main T (1978) Some medical defences against involvement with patients. *J Balint Soc.* **6**.

4 Salinsky J and Sackin P (2000) *What Are You Feeling Doctor?* Radcliffe Medical Press, Oxford.

5 Court SDM (1976) *Fit for the Future.* HMSO, London.

6 Donovan C, Cann P, Kelham I *et al.* (1992) *Health Promotion Clinics: current practices in the NW Thames Region.* Joint Report from the RCGP Clinical and Research Division and RCGP NW Thames Faculty.

7 Neighbour R (1987) *The Inner Consultation.* MTP Press, Lancaster.

8 McWhinney I (1998) *The Physician as Healer.* Proceedings of the Eleventh International Balint Congress, 9–13 September 1998, Oxford, UK.

9 Balint M (1957) *The Doctor, His Patient and the Illness.* Pitman Medical Press, London.

10 Jacobson L, Richardson G, Parry-Langdon N *et al.* (2001) How do teenagers and primary healthcare providers view each other? An overview of key themes. *Br J Gen Pract.* **51**: 811–16.

11 Royal College of General Practitioners and Brook Advisory Centre (2000) *Confidentiality and Young People: a toolkit for general practice, primary care groups and trusts.* Royal College of General Practitioners and Brook Advisory Centre, London.

Chapter 2

A nurse's perspective

Janet Bell

> I think it is essential for young teenagers to go and see a practice nurse every three to six months, male for boys and female for girls. I think this would be very useful for teenagers.
>
> (comment from a young person in the Adolescent Consultations Evaluated (ACE) Project)[1]

Adolescents consult with nurses in general practice on a regular basis. Traditionally, practice nurses provide a range of services that are accessed by all groups of the population. Adolescents may consult for immunisation and vaccination, chronic disease management, contraceptive services, advice and management for minor illnesses.

The role of all nurses working in primary care is changing. Nurses will be providing three core functions:

- first contact – acute assessment, diagnosis, care, treatment and referral
- continuing care – rehabilitation, chronic disease management, palliative care and delivering the National Service Frameworks
- public health/health promotion and protection programmes that improve health and reduce inequalities.[2]

There is no doubt that today practice nurses have an increasing role in primary care, and surveys have reported that nurses enjoy health promotion work and extending their role beyond treatment-room work.[3] Some young people find that access to the practice nurse is easier and less intimidating than access to the GP. There is evidence that, in general practices where there is access to female doctors, young doctors and more nurse time, the teenage pregnancy rate falls to as much as 75% of the expected rate.[4] It is impossible to say what made the greatest contribution to this result, but it is likely that the practice nurses play a significant role. According to the Royal College of Nursing website (October 2003), there are now over 12 500 whole-time-equivalent practice nurses employed in the UK – representing an increase of 40% over the past 10 years.

Personal experience

My continued interest in adolescents and their lifestyles began in 1994 when, as a practice nurse and clinical specialist in family planning in my present five-partner practice in Hertfordshire, I invited 16-year-olds to attend a consultation with me. The aim was to identify some of the health needs of these youngsters. I ran the clinic for six months, and although I was encouraged by the ratio of boys to girls (45% of those attending were boys), I was disappointed by the overall attendance rate (25% of the practice population in this age group). However, this is not unusual for adolescent clinics, with the result that some people consider that designated clinics are not cost-effective.[5] Others take a different view. For example, in 1988 Donovan and McCarthy achieved an attendance rate of more than 50%.[6] Even where the attendance rate is low, the benefit to individuals should not be underestimated.

I am in no doubt as to the benefit of these adolescent consultations, largely because the young people were able to express their concerns. Some of those mentioned were the difficulties they faced because of their parents' marital breakdown, death of a parent or the effects of alcohol abuse in the family. My feeling is that many would be unlikely to discuss such issues at an ordinary surgery appointment. The effects of the consultations can be ongoing. I have noticed that patients whom I see now, who had seen me in the adolescent clinic, value the relationship we started then and may subsequently be more likely to seek help and advice. A specific example of this was demonstrated by a recent consultation of mine. The patient had attended the adolescent clinic as a 16-year-old with her new baby in 1994, and recently came to see me about that same child who is now being bullied at school.

The Adolescent Consultations Evaluated (ACE) Project

This project, a randomised controlled trial, was set up by the University of Hertfordshire in 1997 (under Joy Townsend, who was then Professor of Primary Care), funded by the NHS Executive Eastern Region and by the local research network HertNet.[7] I was invited to become a member of the steering group because of my previous experience of adolescent clinics. The lead researcher, the late Zoe Walker, was inspirational. She motivated the steering group and all of the nurses on the project, throughout the various stages of the project and was appreciative both of our time and of the contributions of the adolescents themselves.

The study was conducted over a period of two years. A total of 1516 adolescents aged 14–15 years from eight practices took part. The aim of the study was to evaluate the effectiveness of inviting adolescents to general practice consultations with a view to changing health behaviour. The intervention was a single consultation with a practice nurse to discuss health concerns and develop plans for healthier lifestyles. The adolescents were seen for follow-up at one and two years.

Significant findings were as follows.

- Many adolescents want to discuss their health concerns.
- A high prevalence of risk behaviour was noted.
- Both physical and mental health concerns were identified and addressed.
- Adolescent health promotion in general practice is well received and may be effective.

All of the nurses involved with the study received two days' training, during which there was a particular emphasis on the importance of confidentiality and consent. The scenarios in the RCGP videos *Trust* and *Clueless* provoked much discussion in small groups. They highlighted dilemmas that nurses face in their everyday work and, although there are rarely clear-cut answers, we felt that we benefited from the opportunity to reflect on these problems. We also learned from our own role playing.

This chapter looks at nurses' consultations with adolescents with the help of the ACE data and my own experiences. The themes discussed here are confidentiality and consent, unpredictability, accommodating attitude and persuading adolescents to talk.

Confidentiality and consent

The Nursing and Midwifery Council states that:[8]

Confidentiality should only be broken in exceptional circumstances and should only occur after careful consideration that you can justify your action ...

Patients have a right to know the standards of confidentiality maintained by those providing their care, and these standards should be made known by the health care professional at the first point of contact ...

A perceived lack of confidentiality has been shown to be associated with avoidance or delay by adolescents in seeking healthcare.[9] The following example illustrates the effects of not clarifying what is meant by confidentiality:

When I went to the doctor's the following day as advised by the nurse, I found that my doctor already knew. She told me that the nurse had told her. However, I thought this appointment was meant to be confidential – if I went again I would not want to talk about personal problems because of this.

Even in our research we encountered difficulties. Two adolescents who were asked to take part had concerns because of relatives who worked in the practices:

I did not go for my appointment because my aunt works at my doctor's and I was worried she would find out stuff I said.

If this questionnaire goes back to the practice, please don't tell my aunt.

An example from my own experience demonstrates that if the adolescent's trust can be gained, they will allow the sharing of information. A young adolescent once presented to me in a severely depressed state. It was a tragic family situation. His father had a progressive disabling disorder, and my patient and his brother had recently been tested to determine whether they carried the gene for this disorder. My patient knew that he did not have the gene but that his brother did, and his brother was already showing signs of the disease. He was able to tell me of his feelings of guilt, anger and sheer hopelessness, and even admitted that he had considered committing suicide by jumping off a local bridge. It was difficult for me, but we were able to discuss the options and available help, and I was relieved that he gave me permission to discuss his problem with his GP.

These situations present the nurse with many dilemmas, and engender a range of emotions which can be so daunting that they can prevent effective communication. However, with specific training, support and experience they can be resolved.

Unpredictability

From my experience as a parent, I know that adolescents act spontaneously. Friday-night activities are decided five minutes before going out. Adolescents seem reluctant to commit themselves to an arrangement more than half an hour beforehand, in case something better turns up. Therefore we should not be surprised that attendance rates for adolescent clinics are relatively low. One boy said to me:

I don't expect you will get many people turning up. I only came because I was nosey.

In the ACE trial, the overall attendance rate was 41%. Attendance rates between the practices involved ranged from 27% to 59%. The nurses who took part in the trial were asked what they felt about the low and unpredictable attendance rates. All of them acknowledged the problem, but they responded in different ways:

You can almost tell by looking at the clinic (list) those who would come. There were a few surprises, but not a lot ...

Rates were lower than I had expected. I assumed that the parents would ensure their offspring attended.

In retrospect I don't think it was too bad – when I ran a previous clinic I had a 25% attendance rate and was told that this was really very good for teenagers.

When asked why the rates varied between practices, one nurse responded:

We're in a very deprived area. The people here will tend to come to the doctor as a sort of reactive thing to something they've got wrong. They don't tend to see health promotion and prevention as something they would ever think about.

Attendance was also thought to depend on:

how accessible the practice is, how well known you are within the practice and if you've been able to have any input beforehand.

Accommodating attitude

The nurses in the ACE project recognised the need for the health professional to adapt to the adolescent's needs:

Be adaptable and flexible. Do not have rigid ideas. All teenagers have different needs.

Listen, enjoy it.

Think about the services available for teenagers – and meet their needs, not the practice's!

Teenagers are an unknown quantity and you never know what they are worried about.

Most adolescents are open, honest and fun. Having three adolescents myself has helped my understanding. I have some idea of what is 'cool' and of the 'in' places. Many practice nurses have adolescents at home, and this helps them not to be affected by attitude, looks and language.

It is not always easy to be accommodating and to respect the adolescent's view. I once phoned a young patient to remind her that she had missed two appointments for her contraceptive injection and that that day was the last day she was protected against pregnancy. She apologised but said she was in the middle of having her hair bleached and would be down as soon as she could!

It is important not to be judgemental or to make assumptions, although this can be difficult, especially when one knows the patient well. I have known Katie since she was about six years old, when she lived with her father and attended the asthma clinic. Now 18 years of age with no permanent home, she has been shunted from one parent to the other for the past six years. She recently met the love of her life, moved in with him, and after he had abused her physically she ran away and made an attempt to commit suicide. With help she regained her self-respect and started talking about college. The last time I saw her she told me that she had moved back in with her former partner. I made a judgemental remark. She looked at me and told me in no uncertain terms that it was none of my business and that she loved him.

For the ACE project we discussed at length how to make the practices 'teenage-friendly'. We highlighted the importance of the attitude of staff, welcoming waiting-rooms, easy access to health professionals, and relevant reading material. I include below some ideas from the adolescents themselves:

> There should be one doctor or nurse who I could see about my problems as a teenager. This is so I could build some sort of trust and they could get to know me as an individual and understand my needs.

> Teenagers feel daunted about talking about their health problems and as a result keep it to themselves. Informing people more fully of what your services involve would help.

Getting adolescents to talk

At a recent workshop on communicating with adolescents, several of the GPs who attended wanted to know how to engage adolescents in dialogue. Experiences shared were of sulky teenagers with their eyes glued to the floor, monosyllabic and grunting, with a parent doing the talking.

Knowing the story behind the adolescent can be an advantage, but I am generally very cautious about mentioning other family members. Adolescents need to be seen and respected as individuals. One young person, with whom it was particularly difficult to communicate seemed troubled when she came to see me. After some time with little progress, I mentioned her mother with caution. The response was immediate. She started talking about how terrible her mother was – always out with her boyfriend, never at home when she came home from school – and she went on in this way for a few minutes. I took a risk in mentioning her mother, but in this case it was the catalyst that allowed us to explore other issues.

Another patient of mine, a 13-year-old girl with diabetes, came to see me recently. She looked amazing, with her hair in high bunches, intricate eye make-up, fishnet tights, a short skirt, layered tops with a fishnet over-shirt and several safety pins about the body. We discussed her love of fashion and how she thought up her ideas. She told me that she wanted to design sexy underwear when she left school. Although this had nothing to do with her diabetes, I felt that this discussion improved our relationship and helped us to work more effectively to control her blood sugar level.

The ACE project encouraged the nurses to confirm the confidentiality policy at the start of each consultation. This was appreciated by the adolescents. A quote from a nurse on the project illustrates the experience of several of us:

> I found that with a lot of them it was more difficult to stop them talking once they had started, rather than getting them to talk, so that was nice.

Conclusion

The adolescents who attended the ACE project reported that they found it useful and helpful. The project provided an opportunity for them to express their health concerns, and for the nurses to identify possible mental and physical problems, and for them both to discuss options for improving lifestyles. The project has provided evidence to support the need for providing adolescents with improved services and for specific training for health professionals.

Practice nurses now have great opportunities to influence local policies through the primary care trusts. Practice nurses are members of primary care boards and are charged with delivering the NHS Plan and National Service Frameworks. In addition, the ACE project has provided us with some good evidence that can be used by practice nurses when negotiating with trusts to provide appropriate teenage services. It is up to us practice nurses to use these facilities to fight for improved services for this important group of patients.

References

1 Walker Z (2001) *The effect on health behaviour of inviting adolescents to a consultation within the general practice setting.* Thesis submitted in partial fulfilment of the requirements of the University of Hertfordshire for the degree of Doctor of Philosophy.
2 Department of Health (2002) *Liberating the Talents. Helping primary care trusts and nurses to deliver the NHS Plan.* Department of Health, London.
3 Robinson H and Robinson A (1993) A survey of practice nurses in Northern Ireland: identifying education and training needs. *Health Education J.* **52**: 208–12.
4 Hippisley-Cox J, Allen J, Pringle M *et al.* (2000) Association between teenage pregnancy rates and the age and sex of general practitioners: cross-sectional survey in Trent 1994–1997. *BMJ.* **320**: 842–5.
5 Churchill R, Allen J, Denman S *et al.* (2000) Do the attitudes and beliefs of young teenagers towards general practice influence actual consultation behaviour? *Br J Gen Pract.* **50**: 953–7.

6   Donovan C and McCarthy P (1988) Is there a place for adolescent screening in general practice? *Health Trends.* **20**: 64–5.

7   Walker Z, Townsend J, Oakley L *et al.* (2002) Health promotion for adolescents in primary care: randomised controlled trial. *BMJ.* **325**: 524–7.

8   United Kingdom Central Council for Nursing, Midwifery and Health Visiting (UKCC) (1996) *Guidelines for Professional Practice.* UKCC, London.

9   Proimos J (1997) Confidentiality issues in the adolescent population. *Curr Opin Pediatr.* **9**: 325–8.

Chapter 3

Reflections of a child and adolescent psychiatrist

Tami Kramer

How I got interested

For almost ten years I have been involved in research concerned with adolescent psychiatric disorder in primary care. I have become increasingly interested in the potential of primary care services to detect and manage distress and psychiatric disorder in adolescents. This interest led to thinking about what happens within the adolescent consultation, and about factors within adolescents, professionals and the health system which facilitate or impair this potential. Attendance at the Difficult Consultations with Adolescents project offered me a unique opportunity to learn about this process and to offer a psychiatrist's perspective on the process.

How did I become interested? My earliest study showed that although very few adolescents (about 2%) present to the GP primarily with emotional or behavioural complaints,[1] rates of psychiatric disorder in those who did attend were far higher than rates in the general population (38% in general practice vs. 20% in the general population). GP identification of 'psychiatric disorder' in our study was poor, despite the fact that the GPs involved had volunteered and were therefore probably particularly interested. When I began to talk to GPs about my findings and to consider how GPs could contribute to this aspect of adolescent care, I became aware of a number of relevant factors. Many GPs believed that adolescents did not use their services. When adolescents did attend, they were often perceived by the GPs as 'difficult'. GPs with an interest in adolescents sometimes expressed discomfort at the idea of using psychiatric 'labels' with what they conceptualised as part of normal adolescence. I began to realise that this area was more complex than my research findings had suggested, and I felt that I needed to consider the context of adolescent consulting more broadly if I was to better understand the potential role of the GP within my area of interest.

The adolescent research background

Research evidence on adolescents in primary care has been accumulating slowly[2] and is described throughout this book. Adolescents do use primary care services,[3,4] despite the long-held misconception that they do not. They have concerns about their physical and emotional health (such as sexually transmitted diseases, contraception, nutrition, acne, weight problems, exercise, arguments with parents, fear of cancer, worry about own death) which they show interest in discussing with their doctor or nurse.[5] They receive shorter consultations from GPs[6] at a time when they are beginning to make decisions about attending for healthcare by themselves.[4] Adolescents have outlined their requirements of primary care, namely confidentiality, staff friendliness, and rapid access to appointments.[7] They want primary care providers to regard them and their health as being of greater importance.[8] Despite the fact that a wide range of health professionals have highlighted the need for services that specifically address the needs of this age group,[9] progress has been slow.[10] The reasons for this are multifaceted, but include the difficulties experienced by professionals when engaging with this work. Jacobson *et al.* have described the need for increased awareness, training, research and resources in order to develop patient-centred services for adolescents.[11]

What I learnt in the Difficult Consultations with Adolescents project

The cases discussed within the project demonstrate many complexities of work with this age group. As a result of participating in the Balint group and reviewing the material generated, a number of themes that contribute to complexity became evident. As with all difficult GP consultations, lack of time is a constraint. This may be even more relevant for adolescents who are just starting to consult on their own or starting to take a lead in the consultation. They will not yet have learned the 'rules of consulting', and may not behave as the GP expects. This apparent non-compliance may generate frustration within the GP (for example, *see* Case 4, page 22). Adolescents may require more help than adults with clearly formulating their problems. Thus silent, vague or tangential presentations may reflect difficulty in finding words rather than a wish to disrupt communication. Many adolescents use emergency appointments rather than booked clinics, adding to the pressure on the GP.[12]

Of course once communication is established the professional needs to be willing to hear and confront the thorny issues as they are raised. These difficulties are well described in previous chapters (for example, *see* page 70 on the GP's experience), and include problems with confidentiality, sex, experimentation with various risks, child protection and family conflicts. The brutal frankness of the adolescent who is communicating has to be accepted and welcomed, however disconcerting it may be. Many cases raised the next dilemma for the professional. Should they respond in the role of the 'protector' or should they facilitate the adolescent's move to autonomy? Just as adolescents will fluctuate between wanting dependence and wishing for independence, the professional will need to oscillate between roles depending on the specific circumstances. On reflection it is no surprise, then, that these consultations are experienced as challenging and filled with an intensity of emotion typical of many normal adolescent experiences. These factors may even contribute to a reluctance to recognise when the patient is an adolescent, and to the relatively shorter consultations.

A general way forward for consultations with adolescents

Despite the complex nature of the cases brought to the group, research has shown that many adolescents are in fact satisfied with what they receive within the consultation.[13] We need to recognise that for many adolescents no change in practice is required, while for some it is.

When cases are more complicated, or generate unease, specific approaches may be helpful. I see two key components. The first concerns *talking to adolescents* generally. Research quoted in this book (*see* Adolescents' views of primary care, on page 65) describes what adolescents want from their GP or practice nurse. Building professionals' confidence in talking to adolescents is essential. It mainly requires increased awareness and practice, although specific training may be helpful. Talking to over 130 adolescent GP attenders helped me to shift my misperception that adolescents are monosyllabic or inarticulate – an experience echoed by others who have focused on this age group (*see* Consulting with adolescents – a nurse's perspective, on page 78).

The second component I see as helpful in making sense of the difficult consultation is the use of a *comprehensive formulation*. This can be applied within a peer discussion group, but can also be used as a template within our thinking to organise ideas.

Formulation structure

Think about:

- the adolescent
    - presenting problem (overt, covert and coincidental problems)
    - presence of illness or disorder (physical or psychological)
    - age and developmental stage (physical, emotional and cognitive)
- functioning within the family (conflicts, changing role, movement towards autonomy)
- functioning within the broader social world (peers, education, work)
- progress of the consultation
- communication with the GP
- outcome of consulting.

The contribution of psychiatric disorder

As mentioned previously, although adolescents almost always present to the GP with physical complaints, a substantial proportion are suffering impairment due to a psychiatric disorder. The relationship between the presence of a psychiatric disorder and consulting is poorly understood (but is evident across the age groups). Our earlier study[1] showed that adolescents with psychiatric disorder experience more impairing physical symptoms, which may lead to increased consulting. This may be because of feelings of vulnerability and a desire for more care. It is important to note that different types of disorder are not equally represented among adolescent GP attenders. There is a preponderance of emotional disorders, with relatively few behavioural disorders. The presence of psychiatric disorder is therefore likely to influence presentation.

Recognition of these emotional disorders could serve a range of functions. It may make overt a hidden morbidity which influences help seeking. Adolescents may be relieved to have their distress recognised, with the potential for specific intervention. They may learn early on that primary care is an access point for help with emotional difficulty, and that emotional complaints are valid in themselves as a reason for presentation. Furthermore, the presence of disorder is associated with greater exposure to health risks, such as drugs and suicidal ideation,[1] presenting an opportunity for prevention.

My suggestion to GPs that they look for psychiatric disorder is sometimes met with opposition. Stigma associated with labelling is cited. Many adolescents may be uneasy about being labelled 'psychiatrically disordered' by the GP, but may be relieved to talk about feeling unhappy or worried. The relief that is evident when their sometimes overwhelming and dreadful feelings are named can be extremely rewarding for the professional. This process does require that the GP provides a bridge within the consultation between the physical and the emotional, which can be challenging and may require specific training. Interviews which we conducted with GPs showed that they vary in the extent to which they feel comfortable talking with teenagers about feelings, and they differ in their beliefs about whether this is their job.

Familiarity with the framework and definitions of psychiatric disorder facilitates the distinction of normal adolescent turmoil and angst from disorder. By definition, the experience of those with disorder differs in either quality or quantity and involves sustained and persistent suffering, usually in association with significant impairment. The mood changes of 'normal adolescence' can be very intense, but are usually very fluctuant and not impairing. Similarly, experimentation with drugs during adolescence is widespread. When this behaviour becomes pervasive, so that it impacts on and impairs other areas of functioning, the behaviour becomes defined as misuse or disorder. Many adolescents feel self-conscious and anxious in social situations, but when this anxiety prevents them from attending school or participating in other activities, it should be recognised as disorder.

Realising the potential of the GP (or primary care) consultation

Within the practical constraints of the ordinary consultation, and noting the unavoidable complexity of a proportion of adolescent presentations, I remain convinced that the consultation is an important opportunity for mental health intervention. On the threshold between childhood and adulthood, adolescents experience disorders characteristic of both of these life phases. Certain common disorders, such as depression and anxiety, are encountered very frequently, and many of these cases will be of mild to moderate severity. On occasion the GP will encounter disorders with more serious consequences, such as severe depression with suicidality, eating disorders, conduct disorders, psychosis or obsessive-compulsive disorder. Usually GPs will need to look for these disorders if they want to find them, although occasionally parents will alert their attention directly. For those interested in detecting this morbidity the checklist below is suggested. Information on specific disorders is given on page 89.

Checklist for detecting psychiatric disorder

- Optimise the context (make the environment adolescent-friendly, offer relevant information leaflets, and see adolescents without a parent present).
- Recognise when you are talking to an adolescent (so that you can recognise the specific features, needs and difficulties within this developmental phase).

- Clarify the boundaries of confidentiality, and clarify them again!
- Seize the opportunity and do what you can within the consultation (the adolescent may not return for some time).
- Know what you are looking for and are most likely to encounter (both developmentally and in terms of psychiatric disorder).
- Be prepared to actively shift the focus of the consultation from the physical to the psychological. For example, use questions like the following.
  - *Other than your acne, how have you been feeling?* or
  - *Do you have any other concerns that I may be able to help you with?*
- Ask questions to elucidate broad areas of relevance, such as the following.
  - *How are things at school/at home/with your friends?*
  - *Are you mainly a happy person or a sad person?*
  In fact very few adolescents see themselves as mainly sad.
- Many adolescents will quickly recognise the relevance of these questions if they are troubled, and those who are not will let you know.
- Where indicated, ask further specific questions (e.g. about depression, thoughts of suicide, eating habits, substance use or psychotic experiences).
- Make relevant leaflets available (*see* Appendix 1).

Remember that *listening and recognising are in themselves therapeutic.*

Specific disorders: ideas on identification and intervention

Depressive disorders

Aids to recognition

The incidence of depressive disorders increases markedly during adolescence, particularly among females. Symptoms are very similar to those in adults (low mood, hopelessness, loss of enjoyment and interest, self-blame, sleep disturbance, appetite disturbance, weight change, and negative thoughts – including those of death and suicide).

Mood must be:

- *pervasive* (i.e. low most of the day), and
- *persistent* over time (on most days for at least two weeks).

Aids to recognition in adolescents

Adolescents may display increased irritability rather than low mood (this results in arguments). Withdrawal from friends and other activities may be the only feature evident to others. Depressive disorders may present as conduct disorder in adolescents with no previous behaviour problems. The adolescent often presents a cheerful façade until you ask specifically, and then tears suddenly become apparent.

Suicidality

Assess suicidality in every depressed adolescent.

Helpful questions include the following.

- *How bad is it when you are at your worst?*
- *Do you think about death or dying? What thoughts do you have?*
- *Do you wish you were not here ... or dead?*
- *When do you have these thoughts? How long do they last?* (Many adolescents have wished they were dead in the heat of an argument, but this does not usually last more than minutes.)
- *Have you ever thought about what you would do? Explain ... What stops you?*

Intervention

Mild to moderate depression (i.e. where symptoms are less intense and impairment is less severe or less widespread)

Adolescents with mild to moderate depression may still be able to attend school and engage in some social activity, although this will require increased effort, achievement at school may be impaired, and social relationships will be less enjoyable.

- Explain to the adolescent what is happening to them (i.e. that they are depressed), what this encompasses and the fact that it is likely to be self-limiting.
- Elucidate any stressors that may be contributing (e.g. bullying, parental depression, etc.). Offer local options for psychotherapeutic intervention.
- Explain the need to return if the condition persists or deteriorates, and offer another appointment.

(*See* Gledhill *et al.*[12] for a description of a GP pilot intervention project.)

Moderate to severe depression (i.e. where symptoms are more intense and impairment is more significant)

Persistent suicidal thoughts or intense hopelessness may be present. Eating and drinking may be reduced. Withdrawal from school, social or family activity may be marked, and psychotic features may be present.

- Explain to the adolescent what is happening to them (i.e. that they are depressed) and what this encompasses.
- Refer them to local mental health provision for assessment and treatment.

Medication

Under 18 years

Prescribing antidepressants to this age group is under debate at present. Specialist assessment before prescribing is currently recommended.

Over 18 years

Consider initiating medication if depression is moderate to severe and if the adolescent is in agreement.

Anxiety disorders

Adolescent anxiety states may resemble those in younger children (i.e. they may include tension and worry about particular situations, separation anxiety, headaches and stomachache). However, at this age, as well as general tension, anxiety states may include *free-floating anxiety* (i.e. a sense of mental unease without focusing on a particular situation), *existential anxiety* (i.e. anxiety about their reality, choices and the meaning of life) and *hypochondriasis* (which is more similar to that seen in adults). Anxieties about personal appearance, attractiveness, loss of friendships and difficulties in socialising are common. Agoraphobia (fear of going out of the home), characterised by fear of being in a situation from which it would be embarrassing or difficult to escape, may begin in adolescence. Obsessive-compulsive disorder is under-recognised, and is characterised by obsessional thoughts and rituals which are impairing. Younger children frequently have rituals that are not impairing. Anxiety states are frequently accompanied by depressive symptoms.

Intervention

Removal or reduction of specific stressors is important. Specific relaxation techniques or other relaxing activities can be very helpful. Brief focused counselling sessions (individual or family) can be used to increase understanding of how anxiety is generated and to improve coping skills.

Eating disorders

Anorexia nervosa

Onset may be pre-adolescent. A parent usually raises concern, and the adolescent will vehemently deny the problem, or may present with other symptoms such as amenorrhoea or constipation. The disorder is characterised by self-induced weight loss (which may be concealed), morbid fear of fat, and misperception of body size. Check the patient's weight using body mass index (BMI) (weight/height^2). A normal BMI is in the range 20–25. Height/weight charts can be misleading in this age group. The index of suspicion should be high. Err on the side of specialist assessment, as detection can be very complex and the consequences of delayed detection can be devastating.

Bulimia nervosa

The incidence of this disorder increases during adolescence. Symptoms include binge eating followed by extreme measures to lose weight (e.g. vomiting, laxative abuse, etc.). It is often accompanied by depressive symptoms. Look for female adolescents with low self-esteem, a history of self-harm, alcohol use, promiscuity, etc. Ask about weight preoccupation, binge eating, self-induced vomiting and laxative use. If in doubt, err on the side of specialist referral.

Substance misuse and dependence

Parents or carers may present with suspicion. They should look for deterioration of function (in school performance and sleep pattern), eating and weight changes, deterioration of personal hygiene and specific physical signs (e.g. alcohol on breath, red eyes), as well as scrutinising peer contacts. In consultation with the adolescent, remain non-judgemental and reiterate confidentiality. Many adolescents will disclose substance use if they know that you will not immediately tell their parents or the police. If you ask without their parents present you will get a more accurate picture.

It is important to recognise that experimentation is widespread, but misuse is less common. Distinguish misuse by assessing whether use is regular and has an impact on any area of functioning (i.e. home, education, peers, work) or whether there is evidence of dependence. Inform the adolescent/parents about local youth drug service provision (this may be within the child and adolescent mental health service, within adult substance misuse services, or the voluntary sector). If the patient is under 16 years of age, remember child protection considerations. Is there evidence of neglect or abuse by the parents or other adults? How is the adolescent funding their substance use? How are they accessing a drug supply? Is the level of adult supervision adequate? Where is substance use taking place? Is the adolescent inappropriately exposed to others who are using substances? (see Appendix 1).

Conduct disorders

Parents will usually present to you, and the adolescent will deny that there is a problem. Conduct disorders are usually preceded by childhood behavioural difficulty. The GP can offer support to the parent and initiate referral to specialist mental health services (which have a role in assessing for treatable comorbidity, such as depression or substance misuse, and may become involved in a network of relevant agencies). The GP can also give parents advice on where else to go for help, particularly if waiting-times for child and adolescent mental health services (CAMHS) are long. Possible relevant agencies include the school or education authority, social services, youth offending team, youth services (e.g. Connexions), parent counselling (either group or individual) or the Young Minds parents' advice line (see page 113).

Psychosis

Parents, carers or the school may first be alerted to difficulties in cases of psychosis. Presentation may be insidious or very acute.

Insidious presentation may be very difficult to recognise in the early stages. It may mimic other conditions or experiences. Presentation could include any of the following: social withdrawal, declining school performance, fluctuating mood, anxiety, acute excitement, or erratic, disturbed or inappropriate behaviour.

Acute presentations are easier to identify. These include abnormal *thoughts* (incoherent, illogical speech), *beliefs* (false beliefs that are impervious to reason and often paranoid), *perceptions* (auditory hallucinations are most common) and *mobility* (abnormal postures or stupor). Remember that the presence of visual hallucinations is more commonly suggestive of an organic pathology such as intoxication or withdrawal from an illicit substance, infection, seizures, etc. Acute presentations should be referred to CAMHS urgently. With a very non-specific insidious presentation, close follow-up over time may be required. If the picture is persistent, with no other obvious cause, refer the adolescent for a specialist opinion.

Conclusion

To conclude, I present a real case vignette that illustrates a very common scenario and demonstrates the views of a typical adolescent attender.

Anna was 16 years old when she gradually began to feel sad and tearful. She withdrew from her friends, whose company she no longer enjoyed, spent much time in her room, and missed school. She lost interest in food and had difficulty sleeping. Increased irritability led to frequent rows with her mother, who started to feel that she did not recognise her daughter any more. Her mother became so frustrated that she yelled 'I wash my hands of you.' These words stuck in Anna's mind. She felt entirely alone, and began to wish that she could disappear or die. She began smoking cannabis every day to block out her thoughts.

During this time she went to see her GP about her acne. She was prescribed a cream, and went home without further discussion. Over the following weeks she describes gradually finding some inner strength to make herself better. She kept telling herself 'You've got to find your old self.' Gradually both she and her relationship with her mother improved, but she did not feel able to tell her mother what it had been like.

When I asked her about her experience of visiting her GP as an adolescent, she replied:

This is the most important time. It's the time you form who you are. When you walk into the surgery you don't know if they see you as a separate person or a little teenager. If you go to the doctor and they dismiss you, it's terrible. To them concerns about appearance are so minor; to you it's a big thing.'

References

1 Kramer T and Garralda ME (1998) Adolescents in primary care: the contribution of psychiatric disorder. *Br J Psychiatry*. **173**: 508–13.

2 Walker ZA and Townsend J (1999) The role of general practice in promoting teenage health: a review of the literature. *Fam Pract*. **16**: 164–72.

3 Department of Health (1992) *General Household Survey*. HMSO, London.

4 Balding J (1994) *Young People in 1993*. HEA Schools Health Education Unit, University of Exeter, Exeter.

5 Epstein R, Rice P and Wallace P (1989) Teenagers' health concerns: implications for primary health care professionals. *J R Coll Gen Pract*. **39**: 247–9.

6 Jacobson L, Wilkinson C and Owen P (1994) Is the potential of teenage consultations being missed? A study of consultation times in primary care. *Fam Pract*. **11**: 296–9.

7 Donovan C, Mellanby AR, Jacobson LD *et al.* for the RCGP Adolescent Working Party (1997) Teenagers' views on the general practice consultation and provision of contraception. *Br J Gen Pract*. **47**: 715–18.

8 Jacobson L, Richardson G, Parry-Langdon N *et al.* (2001) How do teenagers and primary healthcare providers view each other? An overview of key themes. *Br J Gen Pract*. **51**: 811–16.

9 Macfarlane A and McPherson A (1995) Primary health care and adolescence. *BMJ*. **311**: 825–6.

10 Viner R and Macfarlane A (2000) Provision of age-appropriate health services for young people has been ignored. *BMJ*. **321**: 1022.

11 Jacobson L, Churchill R, Donovan C *et al.* for the RCGP Adolescent Working Party (2002) Tackling teenage turmoil: primary care recognition and management of mental ill health during adolescence. *Fam Pract.* **19**: 401–9.

12 Gledhill J, Kramer T, Iliffe S *et al.* (2003) Training general practitioners in the identification and management of adolescent depression within the consultation: a feasibility study. *J Adolesc.* **26**: 245–50.

13 Jacobson LD, Mellanby AR, Donovan C *et al.* for the RCGP Adolescent Party (2000) Teenagers' views on general practice consultations and other medical advice. *Fam Pract.* **17**: 156–8.

Chapter 4

What do young people tell ChildLine about their doctors?

Sheila R Cross

ChildLine is a telephone helpline for children and young people. Most people associate it with child abuse and bullying, and it is true that together with family problems these constitute the greater part of ChildLine's work. A number of other problems contribute a small percentage of the total calls, but because the numbers calling are so large, these small percentages represent large numbers of calls. They include about 5000 calls each year about physical and mental health problems. From the computerised call summaries and the original case notes we can learn a great deal about what young people are saying.

I came to ChildLine as a volunteer telephone counsellor in 1991 when I was nearing retirement. As a full-time paediatrician in a district general hospital, the majority of my patients had been under 12 years of age, and most of my teenage patients had grown up in the paediatric clinic rather than coming as new referrals. I had often felt at a loss with adolescents. As they sat beside their mothers (rarely their fathers), their faces giving nothing away, I used to wonder what they were thinking. It seemed likely that they took a dim view of me, did not want to be there, and did not have much hope that I could solve their problems. If I saw them alone, they rarely confided in me and almost certainly expected me to report back to their parent. Working at ChildLine gave me a privileged insight into young people's problems, their concern for their parents, their poor view of themselves and much else. I also heard their rage and learned a new vocabulary. There was no dramatic change in my clinic as a result of what I learned at ChildLine – teenagers did not recognise the change in me and did not more eagerly seek to trust me with their confidences – but I felt more at ease, less threatened, and now often had some idea of their unspoken concerns.

At ChildLine I had a lot to learn. The medical pattern of work was second nature to me, but the ability to define a problem, explain and prescribe a plan of action all within a 20-minute consultation was now hopelessly inappropriate. I learned to listen and allow young people time to work out their own solutions. Meanwhile my colleagues at ChildLine were glad to be able to ask me for explanations of illnesses and symptoms voiced by their clients, and sometimes for help in understanding the reported words of doctors.

My interest in young people was heightened and in 1998 I wrote the report '*I Know You're Not a Doctor But ...*'. *Children calling ChildLine about health.*[1] This report was based on a study of 792 calls about a wide variety of health problems. When invited to contribute this chapter I looked at a further 100 more recent call summaries to see whether there was any change in emphasis, but found very little difference. I had initially expected anger and complaints about doctors, but found little. Perhaps there is a depressing impression that young people do not really expect very much from their doctor. Nevertheless, there is much of interest and, I hope, of use in these unsolicited comments. The quotations in this chapter are drawn both from the report and from the more recent sample. The details of each individual have been altered in order to protect the confidentiality of information provided by all callers.

Confidentiality

Confidentiality remains a major concern, and with good reason. There has been a change in young people's expectations. Whereas in the past they often asked whether they could expect their doctor to keep what they told him or her confidential, it seems that they now expect it as their right. There are many who are disappointed and angry.

Robert

Robert went to see his GP because he was drinking too much. There were other problems at home and his GP called in social services. Although Robert was finding his social worker very helpful, he said about his doctor:

I'm very angry. He's supposed to keep things confidential.

Robert was not being abused, and from his account it is difficult to understand why the GP did not discuss the referral with him.

Gillian

Gillian, aged 17 years, was depressed and had consulted her GP about counselling or a referral to a psychiatrist. Her mother was dead. The GP had spoken with Gillian's father, and the resulting upheaval had ended in Gillian being thrown out of her home. She had gone to live with her grandmother, but had had to move school and was far from her friends.

John

John had confided in his GP and been astonished to learn that his doctor had subsequently spoken with his father, who felt that he had been unjustly criticised by John. John said:

I didn't tell him he could talk to Dad, and I didn't say I thought it was Dad's fault, but Dad won't believe me.

There is often great difficulty for young people who live in small communities:

I can't tell my GP. He plays golf with my Dad.

The receptionist is Mum's best friend.

Doctors also need to consider the needs of their own children.

> **Daphne**
>
> Daphne wanted to see a woman doctor about contraception. The counsellor asked:
>
> Is there a woman in the practice?
>
> Yes [said Daphne], my mother.

There are also complaints about doctors 'telling the school'. It is not usually clear whether this means the education staff or the school health staff, and almost certainly to the caller they are one and the same. The doctor may think that this is constructive and helpful action, but callers certainly resent this sharing of information without their consent.

One outraged caller told us that his doctor had given medical information in a reference to an employment agency without consent.

Respect

It is clear in many calls to ChildLine that young people, like adults, harbour secret fears about their health. When they find the courage to tell someone about these anxieties, they need to feel that they are being taken seriously. Reading the records, it is possible to detect that the doctor intended reassurance but in fact callers were not reassured by hearing their symptoms dismissed.

> **Peter**
>
> Peter told us he had abdominal pain and had asked his doctor for an X-ray.
> She just said 'You don't need one.'
> He did not seem to have been given any explanation, and could not understand how the doctor could be so sure of this. He was left with the fear that he had cancer.

> **Anne**
>
> A girl who had experimented with drugs a week previously now had symptoms that frightened her. She plucked up courage to phone her doctor.
> He just said:
>
> That's nothing to do with it.

> **Tracy**
>
> Tracy, in her early teens, felt that she was growing excess body hair.
> The doctor just said:
>
> It's all in the mind.

As doctors we can hear the reassurance intended in these responses, but perhaps the use of the word 'just' sums up the feeling that the young people were left with. They did not feel that their symptoms – real or imagined – had been given sufficient attention. They wanted explanations, and perhaps they also needed to feel that they themselves were worthy of an explanation.

Doctors, like other adults, reassure themselves (but not their patients) with the platitude 'You'll grow out of it.' This may or may not be true – many ills do go away by themselves at all ages – but it is no help to the teenager who wets the bed or the boy with a depression that seems unending.

One boy who was worried about his smoking was told by his GP 'Go away and stop wasting my time.' Would a doctor, however provoked, feel able to speak to an adult patient like that?

Explanation

Callers often say that they are worried by what they have been told and want an explanation. They ring ChildLine because it is easier to ask an unknown listener what the doctor meant than to go back to the surgery.

Mitali

Mitali was having problems with her lifestyle.
    She told us:

    The doctor says I am in a 'dangerous state'. I don't know what he means.

We might guess what the doctor meant. Mitali knew that she wanted to change things but had no idea what he meant. Was she going to die? How soon? Did he mean the police would be involved?

Lee

Lee had been sent for blood tests. He did not know what they were for.

    Does he think I've got AIDS? Can I refuse?

Jim

A courageous teenager felt that his parents had made a wrong decision about his treatment. He had been to the doctor by himself.

    He said he agreed with me, but I don't know whether he is going to do anything. He didn't say.

Young people are often excluded from discussions about the illness of other family members. They are fearful and may be left feeling responsible for the illness. Much distress might be avoided if their need could be recognised and shown to the family.

> **Will**
>
> Will had left home. He was called back because his father was ill, and he was left feeling that the illness was all his (Will's) fault. No one had told him what was wrong with his father. It had not occurred to him that he could ask the family doctor (who could seek permission from the father to tell him).

Young people not only feel responsible for their parents, but may also be forced by circumstances into the role of responsible adult. It is hard when the doctor chooses to ignore this situation.

> I have told the doctor that my mother is too depressed to get up in the morning. He says he can't do anything unless she comes to see me herself.

> I live with my Nan. She is missing Grandad. She won't eat and is sick a lot. The doctor says he needs to talk to a grown-up, but there isn't anyone.

A rare note of anger is sometimes heard:

> My sister's very depressed. The doctor won't listen to me. He's given her sleeping tablets. How stupid can you get?

Control

Young people, in common with most adults, want to feel in control of their lives. All too often illness means forfeiting control to the doctor. More than one caller on maintenance for chronic illnesses told us of taking 'unofficial control'. They had not been able to share this feeling with the doctor, who was seen as in authority and demanding obedience:

> I vary the dose to feel in control.

Sometimes it seems that the doctor is being more dogmatic than is necessary, and the patient rings ChildLine as if to appeal to a different authority:

> He said I must tell my parents.

> He said I must decide today whether to have an abortion or keep it.

These young people felt that they were in an impasse, yet it did not take more than one call to ChildLine to help them to look at options and if necessary accept the inevitable with a feeling that they were making their own decisions.

Getting it right

We know that even when things are going well, children and young people ring ChildLine to talk to an independent listener, and there are plenty of callers who regard their doctor as an ally.

> My doctor was shocked by the bruises and called social services.

> My doctor said it's the bullying that's making me ill, and she's written to the school.

Callers describing their depression commonly talk of going to the doctor and being referred to a counsellor, or prescribed antidepressants, or followed up regularly, even though some may find no improvement.

> He's ever so nice and sees me every week, but it's not doing any good.

Some give accounts of consultations with doctors who have taken time to listen and given advice in ways which have been accepted. A 14-year-old told us:

> It's awful at home. I want to run away. I've been to the doctor but he says he doesn't think I'm quite strong enough to live alone yet.

Jeff

Jeff was threatened by an abusing uncle who was out looking for him. Talking from a phone box, Jeff told us that the doctor's surgery would be a safe place to run to. We learned later that he had reached the surgery, been warmly cared for by the receptionist and, after phone calls by the doctor, had been taken into safety.

Conclusion

Talking spontaneously and knowing that they are speaking in confidence, the young people who call ChildLine offer us valuable insights if we are willing to hear them. It seems that young people only want from their doctor the things we all want – to be heard, to be respected, and to be treated kindly and in confidence. Is it too much to hope that they should all, like Jeff, see their doctor's surgery as a 'safe place' to seek help?

Reference

1   Cross S (1998) 'I Know You're Not a Doctor But ...'. Children calling ChildLine about health. ChildLine, London.

Part 5

Conclusions

The reality that the needs of many adolescents are not being met is shown by the UK's high rates of teenage suicide and pregnancy, substance misuse, mental health problems and sexually transmitted disease. It is also reflected in the mortality figures for this age group (which have not changed in the last 10 years), the quality of care for many chronic conditions, the lack of effective prevention and the need for increased health promotion. For humanitarian reasons, and also in an ageing society for economic reasons, our services for patients in this age group need to be improved so that adolescents can be given more support to help them with their problems, thus enabling more young people to have a chance to grow into effective adults, parents and wealth creators.

Those who are looking to improve primary care services for adolescents need to consider three parameters:

- outcome
- structure
- process.

There is a danger in the belief that improving structure alone will be sufficient. This project reinforces the fact that outcome is dependent on both structure and process, both of which depend on sufficient resources. More attention needs to be paid to the process that the patient has to undergo in order to access professional help, and to doctor–patient consultations. GPs need the resources and skills to be able to develop a trusting relationship with their adolescent patients, preferably in the early years of adolescence before major problems arise – for example, by seeing them on their own for some of the consultation, or by running an adolescent clinic. More and better training in adolescent communication skills for all professionals, more effective continuity of care and improved back-up services in secondary care may also ease the discomfort and difficulties experienced by both parties in some of the more sensitive consultations.

This project, which discusses only a handful of consultations, has raised important issues that need to be investigated further. Although they are subjective accounts of difficulties experienced in the process of consulting with some adolescent patients by some professionals, the 'themes' identified are areas that call for further research, and many of these themes need to be included in training programmes.

The consultations presented in this project were classified as 'difficult' by the doctors. Although many of the issues raised are also likely to be of concern to adolescents, a group of adolescents might identify different problems for discussion. Indeed some of the cases presented here may not have been classified as difficult by the adolescent involved, especially the cases where the doctor was left feeling uneasy even though the patient had apparently received what they requested (for example, see Cases A, 6 and 8).

Problems in consultations may arise because of factors in the doctor, the reason for the consultation, the patient or the system. For example, the doctor may lack adequate perception or communication skills, the reason for the consultation may be unclear, the patient may be too embarrassed to communicate effectively, the system may not provide sufficient time, and continuity of care may be impossible. These challenges are compounded by the developmental process of adolescence, by the high expectations placed on primary care professionals by patients, their families, schools, society and the professionals themselves, and by the lack of available sources of support from secondary care. The aims of this project consultations were twofold – firstly, to make interactions more productive for the patient and, secondly, to make them less stressful for the professional. In this context, methods of providing more training, time and support/supervision (in the psychotherapeutic sense) for professionals stand out as areas for further consideration. Those who participated in this project benefited from discussing difficult consultations which had left them with feelings that they had not previously shared with colleagues, in some cases for months.

The difficulty of balancing the needs of adolescent patients with those of other patients in each surgery was not discussed to any great extent by the group, but the authors feel that it is worthy of further consideration, especially within the constraints of relatively short consultation times in primary care. The trend within the NHS is to emphasise the need to provide quality services, but the definition of quality is becoming increasingly reliant on activities that can be measured (e.g. statistics for immunisation, cervical smears, blood pressure and smoking status). We fear that the need for primary care to demonstrate these measurable outcomes militates against the quality which we feel will result from improving the consultation itself. Although it is hard to measure, the improvement in quality of a consultation is recognised as important by patients and doctors, as demonstrated by the work of Jacobson *et al.*[1] Most adolescent patients, we believe, are looking for an effective and trusting relationship with their doctor or nurse – someone who will listen to them empathetically, who will spend time reflecting on their problems and who will 'be there' for them if they choose to return. Most adolescents need this in addition to effective, evidence-based and up-to-date clinical and preventive care. The group tacitly recognised that quality in this context may not be something which can be easily measured, but it can be described. It is becoming increasingly evident that health professionals who reflect on their interactions, as they did in this project, can learn from them and subsequently improve the quality of their practice.

This project focused on *difficult* consultations. However, the group agreed that many consultations with adolescents are not difficult. Easy and productive consultations may also provide clues as to how young people might be better helped by the primary care services. The experiences of a wider sample of health professionals and adolescents might help to increase our understanding of some of the issues raised in this project. Further research into both difficult and satisfactory adolescent consultations within and beyond primary care is needed in order to determine how widespread the themes identified in this project are in today's consultations.

Most adolescents obtain their greatest support from their parents and extended families, but there are many others in schools, colleges and the wider community who can also provide much-needed support, both formally and informally (some of the organisations are listed in Appendix 1). The group discussions emphasised the need for all those working on behalf of adolescents to find ways of communicating more effectively and to increase their learning about each other's roles, so that they can work together to help young people to take increasing responsibility for their own physical and mental health and enable them to use the services appropriately.

Perhaps the greatest contribution of this project is that it describes real-life consultations in which the health professionals had experienced difficulties. It was their courage in revealing and discussing their concerns, mistakes and regrets which enabled the work to take place. We hope that this will stimulate others to reflect on their consultations, and that some will undertake further research along these lines.

Reference

1 Jacobson L, Richardson G, Parry-Langdon N *et al.* (2001) How do teenagers and primary healthcare providers view each other? An overview of key themes. *Br J Gen Pract.* **51:** 811–16.

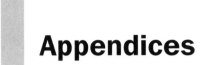

Appendices

Appendix 1

Resources

Sources of information for professionals wishing to study this subject further

Books

- Coleman and J Schofield J (2003) *Key Data on Adolescence* (4e). Trust for the Study of Adolescence, Brighton.

- Coleman J and Hendry L (1999) *The Nature of Adolescence* (3e). Routledge, London.

- Dogra N, Parkin A, Gale F and Frake C (2002) *A Multi-Disciplinary Handbook of Child and Adolescent Mental Health for Frontline Professionals.* Jessica Kingsley, London.

- Gowers S (ed.) (2001) *Adolescent Psychiatry in Clinical Practice.* Arnold, London.

- Graham P, Verhulst F and Turk J (1999) *Child Psychiatry: a developmental approach* (3e). Oxford University Press, Oxford.

- Salinsky J (2001) *What are You Feeling, Doctor? Identifying and avoiding defensive patterns in the consultation.* Radcliffe Medical Press, Oxford.

- Silverman J and Kurtz S (1998) *Skills for Communicating with Patients.* Radcliffe Medical Press, Oxford.

Factsheets

- *Surviving Adolescence.*
  Gives a good overview of problems in adolescence.
  Available from the Royal College of Psychiatrists or from their website: www.rcpsych.ac.uk/info/help/adol/index.htm

- *Mental Health and Growing Up: factsheets for parents, teachers and young people.*
  Includes 36 different factsheets on different conditions and family problems.
  Available from the Royal College of Psychiatrists or from their website: www.rcpsych.ac.uk/info/mhgu/index.htm

Sources of general information suitable for parents, young people and professionals (could be used in the consultation)

- McConville B (2002) *Where to Look for Help: a guide for parents and carers of teenagers.* TSA Ltd, Brighton.
  Available from the Trust for the Study of Adolescence; Tel: 01273 693311
  Excellent small ringfile that provides a guide to most organisations that help young people. Should be available in every surgery. £16.45 + p & p, £10 to parents.

- **Get Connected**
  Tel: 0808 808 4994 (1pm to 11pm)
  Website: www.getconnected.org.uk
  Free helpline that will put you through to the organisation that will best be able to help with whatever your problem is.

- **Teenage Health Freak**
  Website: www.teenagehealthfreak.co and www.doctorann.org
  Answers questions you would not dare ask your doctor – run by the authors of *Diary of a Teenage Health Freak*, Dr Ann McPherson and Dr Aidan Macfarlane.

- **Muslim Women's Help Line**
  Tel: 020 8904 8193
  Many young Muslim women call this helpline for advice about a wide range of problems.

Material that might be of help when teaching this subject

Videos concerning young people in contact with primary healthcare services. Ten minutes long, each showing four short interviews, designed to stimulate discussions on methods of improving surgery services for young people. *Clueless* covers the role of the receptionist, practice nurse and general practitioner, *Trust* covers aspects of confidentiality relevant to members of the primary care team.

Available from the Royal College of General Practitioners; Tel: 020 7581 3232 or from Chris Donovan; Tel: 020 8458 4526. Price: £7.00 + p & p.

- **TSA Ltd**
  Tapewise Ltd
  23 New Road
  Brighton
  East Sussex
  BN1 1WZ
  Tel: 01273 693311
  This organisation has produced a series of audiotapes and booklets about adolescence and common problems, called *Tapes for Teenagers*. The series was devised by Dr John Coleman of the Trust for the Study of Adolescence.

- *Bridging the Gaps: Health Care for Adolescents.* June 2003. Royal College of Paediatrics and Child Health.
  Thoughts of a committee representing most of the Royal Medical Colleges on how to improve medical services for adolescents. Divided into problems of primary and secondary care.

- *Confidentiality and Young People: A toolkit for general practice, primary care groups and trusts.* Endorsed by the Royal College of General Practitioners, the British Medical Association, the Royal College of Nursing and the Medical Defence Union. Available from the Department of Health.

- Hughes T, Garralda ME and Tylee A (1994) *Child Mental Health Problems.* A booklet and video on child psychiatric problems for general practitioners. Available from the Department of Child and Adolescent Psychiatry, Paddington Green; Tel: 020 7886 1145.

- McPherson A, Macfarlane A and Donovan C (2002) *Healthcare of Young People: promotion in primary care.* Radcliffe Medical Press, Oxford.

Individual sources of help

There are many national voluntary bodies that can help adolescents, some are listed below. Every surgery should have a comprehensive list of local and national sources of help to hand out when appropriate as an extension of the consultation.

- **Al Anon**
  61 Great Dover Street
  London
  SE1 4YF
  Helpline: 020 7403 0888 (7 days a week, 10am–10pm)
  Website: www.hexnet.co.uk/alanon
  Help with drink, drugs and addiction. Nine hundred groups across the UK. They believe in self-help and support for families of problem drinkers. Runs Alateen for young people between 12 and 20 years of age.

- **Anti-Bullying Campaign**
  10 Borough High Street
  London
  SE1 9QQ
  Tel: 020 7378 1446

- **Brent Adolescent Centre**
  Johnston House
  51 Winchester Avenue
  London
  NW6 7TT
  Tel: 020 7328 0918

14–21 year olds can self-refer or be referred by their GP or social worker for emotional/ suicidal problems and drug and alcohol difficulties in and around Brent. They are seen for free assessment within a week or two by well-trained staff.

- **British Association for Counselling**
  1 Regent Place
  Rugby
  TZ21 2PJ
  Tel: 01788 578328
  Will send you a list of counsellors in your area experienced in counselling young people.

- **British Agencies for Adoption and Fostering**
  Skyline House
  200 Union Street
  London
  SE1 0LX
  Tel: 020 7593 2000

- **Brook Advisory Centre**
  233 Tottenham Court Road
  London
  W1 9AE
  Tel: 020 7713 9000
  Provides free, confidential sex advice and contraception for young people including those under 16 years. Has many local centres and provide many publications.

- **ChildLine**
  Freepost 1111
  London
  N1 0BR
  Tel: 0800 1111
  Website: www.childline.org.uk/
  A free national helpline for children in trouble or danger. It provides a confidential counselling service 24 hours a day.

- **Child Psychotherapy Trust**
  Star House
  104–8 Grafton Road
  London
  NW5 4BD
  Tel: 020 7284 1355

- **Cystic Fibrosis Trust**
  27 Spencer Street
  Carlisle
  CA1 1BE
  Tel: 01228 597 405

- **Eating Disorders Association**
  Sackville Place
  44 Magdalen Street
  Norwich
  NR3 1JU
  Youth helpline: 01603 765050

- **First Key (National Leaving Care Advisory Service)**
  Tel: 0113 244 3898

- **It's Not Your Fault**
  Gives support and advice to young people whose parents are divorcing or separating.
  Website: www.itsnotyourfault.org

- **Lesbian and Gay Switchboard**
  Helpline: 020 7837 7324 (24 hours)
  Website: www.llgs.org.uk
  Advice, information and a listening ear for lesbian and gay people and concerned parents.

- **Manic Depression Fellowship**
  Castleworks
  21 St George's Road
  London
  SE1 6ES
  Tel: 020 7793 2600

- **Message Home**
  Helpline: 0800 700 740
  Enables those who have run away to leave a message for parents or social workers.

- **MIND Information Line**
  Tel: 020 8522 1728

- **NHS Health Information**
  Tel: 0800 665544

- **NSPCC (National Society for the Prevention of Cruelty to Children)**
  42 Curtain Road
  London
  EC2A 3NH
  Tel: 020 7825 2500
  Helpline: 0800 800 500

- **Nat Council for One-Parent Families**
  Promotes welfare of lone parents and families. Provides financial advice and useful handouts.
  Free helpline: 0800 018 5026
  Website: www.oneparentfamilies.org.uk

- Parentline Plus
  Tel: 0808 800 2222
  Website: www.parentlineplus.org.uk/
  A registered charity that offers support to anyone parenting a child (the child's parents, step-parents, grandparents or foster parents).

- Rape Crisis Centre
  PO Box 69
  London
  WC1 9NJ
  Tel: 020 7837 1600 (24 hours)

- RSSPCC (Royal Scottish Society for the Prevention of Cruelty to Children)
  Melville House
  41 Polwarth Terrace
  Edinburgh
  EH11 1NU
  Tel: 0131 337 8539

- The Samaritans
  10 The Grove
  Slough
  SL1 1QP
  Tel: 08457 909090 in the UK (1850 609090 in Eire), or look for the number of your local branch in the phone directory
  The Samaritans is a registered charity that provides confidential emotional support for any person who is suicidal or despairing. It also increases public awareness of issues relating to suicide and depression.

- Survivors of Sexual Abuse
  Tel: 020 8890 4732

- Trust for the Study of Adolescence
  23 New Road
  Brighton
  East Sussex
  BN1 1WZ
  Tel: 01273 693311
  Publications department has books and games suitable for adolescents. Does much research on adolescent problems and produces *Key Data on Adolescence*, updated every two years.

- **Young Minds**
  102–108 Clerkenwell Road
  London
  EC1M 5SA
  Tel: 020 7336 8445
  Parents' Information Service: 0800 018 2138 (Monday/Friday 10am–1pm; Tuesday/Wednesday/Thursday 1pm–4pm).
  Website: www.youngminds.org.uk
  Young Minds is a national charity that promotes the mental health of children and young people. Resources available online include leaflets, resource sheets, Young Minds publications, the Young Minds magazine and links to other relevant websites.

As well as organisations it is helpful to have pamphlets available giving information on subjects like drugs or eating disorders, etc. to hand out during the consultation. The local Health Promotion Unit or one of the above organisations will provide these. National lists of local units are available from Health Education Authority library and information service; Tel: 020 7383 5833.

Some professionals have, in addition to pamphlets, samples of appropriate books to show to patients during the consultation. We give some examples below but there are many more, all obtainable from Trust for the Study of Adolescence. Tel: 01273 693 311.

- Wiseguide Series (*Drinking, Bullying, Self-Esteem, Sex*)
  Matthew Wyman, Hodders Childrens Books 2002. Price: £5.99.

- *The Smart Girls Guide to Boys*
  Maria Coole, Piccadily Press 2000. Price: £5.99.

- *Everything You Ever Wanted to Ask About …*
  Willies and Other Boys' Bits
  Tricia Kreitman, Neil Simpson, Rosemary Jones. Piccadily Press 2002. Price: £6.99.
  This really useful book is based on what boys have said and really want to know. It provides facts about this mysterious and unpredictable part of their anatomy.

- *Everything You Ever Wanted to Ask About …*
  Periods
  Tricia Kreitman, Neil Simpson, Rosemary Jones. Piccadily Press 2002. Price: £5.99.

- *Self-Harm: Young People Speaking Out*
  Sheffield City Council Women's Committee and TSA 2001. Price: £2.00
  Excellent booklet written by young people who self-harm, offering advice on coping strategies.

Appendix 2

The history of the Balint group

'Balint' refers to Michael Balint, a Hungarian psychoanalyst who, together with his third wife, Enid, started groups for GPs in the 1950s.

Michael Balint, the son of a GP, was born in Budapest in 1896. He became a medical student at the age of 16 years, but his studies were interrupted by World War One when he joined the army and served on the Russian and Italian fronts. However, after being wounded he resumed his studies in his native Budapest, and obtained his doctorate in 1920. Initially he wanted to be a biochemist, but after hearing Freud speak at conferences and reading *The Interpretation of Dreams*, he developed an increasing interest in psychoanalysis. This was encouraged by his first wife, Alice Szekely-Kovacs, who was herself an analyst. He subsequently trained as a psychoanalyst, his trainer and mentor being Sandor Ferenczi, who was a contemporary of Freud, but of the Hungarian School, which was more eclectic than the Viennese. Balint worked as an analyst in Budapest until 1939 when, because he was Jewish, he was obliged to leave Hungary and move to Manchester with his wife and son as a refugee. Sadly, Alice died the same year. Balint remarried soon afterwards, but his second marriage, to Edna, was brief and ended in divorce. He had moved to London, working initially in child guidance clinics until he was appointed to the Tavistock Clinic. There he met (and in 1949 married) Enid Echoltz (née Albu), who was a social worker and marriage guidance counsellor, and they developed their innovative groups for GPs together.

The Balints began their groups shortly after the inception of the National Health Service, when for the first time free healthcare for all had been introduced, and as a result GPs' surgeries were flooded with patients with high expectations. The GPs, who at that time had had no specific training for general practice, were ill-equipped to deal with unclear diagnoses, particularly of emotional problems in an atmosphere where patients believed that there was now a cure for all of their ills.

Balint was one of the first to recognise the value of the consultation itself as a therapeutic tool. As an analyst he realised that what happened psychologically between the doctor and the patient was significant, although this was not discussed in medical textbooks of the day. This was before the days of consultation analysis and communications skills training, although there were of course doctors who recognised the importance of listening to their patients. The Balints advertised for doctors to join a group for 'training and research' to study the doctor–patient relationship. The traditional Balint group was born and the outcome of this first group was Balint's seminal work, *The Doctor, his Patient and the Illness*,[1] which was published in 1957.

Postgraduate training for general practice was instituted in the early 1970s, and was greatly facilitated by the publication of the book *The Future General Practitioner: Learning and Teaching*.[2] It is of interest to note that half of the authors had been in a Balint group, and there is no doubt that this led to the almost universal use of the small group in GP training. Balint's influence is evident even in the subtitle of the book, 'learning and teaching', with the then revolutionary idea that these took place simultaneously for both the pupil and the teacher.

The Balints were at pains to avoid a teacher–pupil relationship in the groups:

> What we aimed at was a free give-and-take atmosphere in which everyone could bring up his problems in the hope of getting some light on them from the experience of others.

References

1 Balint M (1957) *The Doctor, his Patient and the Illness.* Pitman Medical Press, London.
2 Horder J, Byrne P, Freeling P *et al.* (1972) *The Future General Practitioner: learning and teaching.* Royal College of General Practitioners, London.

Child protection issues and sexual health services

Karen E Rogstad and Helen King

The following is a paper submitted to the Royal College of Paediatrics and Child Health (RCPCH) working party on the responsibilities of paediatricians in child protection cases with regard to confidentiality, and we suggest that readers look at the final guidelines of the RCPCH when they are published. An editorial based on and containing large portions of this paper has already been published:

- Rosgrad K and King H (2003) Child protection issues and sexual health services in the UK. *J Fam Plan Reprod Health Care*. **29**: 182–3.

  There are difficulties in providing sexual health services to young people, as they are entitled to the same degree of confidentiality as adults[1–3] and can consent to examination and treatment if Fraser (Gillick) competent.[4] However, according to the law their sexual activity may be defined as unlawful either due to their age, the age of their partner or if they are involved in prostitution. Sexual activity is particularly an issue for the under-13s in that they can be judged Fraser competent to consent to examination and treatment but are regarded as incapable of consenting to sexual activity, requiring referral to Child Protection services or the police. The care of children and young people is guided by the standards laid down in statute for sexually transmitted disease (STD) services,[5] the Children Act 1989,[6] the European Convention on Human Rights[7] and the Human Rights Act.[8] This will be further affected by the Sexual Offences Bill if this becomes law,[9] which defines any penetrative sexual activity under the age of 13 years as rape and any sexual activity between an adult aged 18 years or over with a child under 16 years as an offence with a maximum sentence of 14 years' imprisonment. The medical profession has raised concerns about this, and a supplement has been added stating that

  a person acts for the protection of a child if he acts for the purpose of (a) protecting the child from sexually transmitted infection, (b) protecting the physical safety of a child, or (c) preventing a child from becoming pregnant, and not for the purpose of causing or encouraging the activity constituting the offence within subsection (1)(b) or the child's participation in it.

  That such young people are sexually active is considered undesirable, but this is the reality in some areas of the country. In some places it is not unusual for girls of 12 years with partners of 13 or 14 years who appear not to be 'at risk' other than from pregnancy and STIs to access services. This poses different problems for health professionals [seeing them], and can result in conflict between professional codes of confidentiality, the expectations of the client/young person, a young person's needs for sexual health services and Child Protection guidance. National guidelines have been produced on the management of suspected sexually transmitted diseases in children and young people which discuss this in more detail.[10] .... Doctors providing these services cannot and should not ignore the child protection issues for these young people. However, they must also consider the needs and rights of the young person for confidential and appropriate medical care. If a service is not seen to be confidential then it is possible either that it will not be accessed or that those attending will not be honest about their age, sexual activity or disclose abuse or exploitation. This would have catastrophic health implications and mean that abuse/exploitation would go unrecognised and the opportunity for supporting the young person and intervening to stop the abuse/exploitation would be lost. Currently many contraceptive services provide a confidentiality statement which specifies that if abuse is disclosed this will be reported. The effect of such statements on a young person's willingness to then disclose important information about sexual abuse/exploitation and about their partner for contact tracing purposes is unknown ...

Doctors and nurses ... need to be able to discuss clients without initial disclosure of names. The distinction between the need for advice/discussion and referral is an important one. The effect of the Climbie Enquiry[11] on information sharing by sexual health services is currently unknown. If referral is necessary the child's consent should be obtained, and if refused it may be possible to work with the young person over a period of time in order to obtain consent, unless there is evidence of immediate danger or risk to another child. If disclosure is refused they should be made aware of the referral except in exceptional circumstances. It is essential that every case is dealt with on an individual basis, and that close collaboration between services exists ...

When a boy or girl is working or suspected of working in prostitution, they need referral for STI screening, hepatitis B vaccination and advice on safer sexual practices. If samples are taken for STI testing in sexual abuse victims, then a 'chain of evidence' form should be used for forensic purposes. National guidelines on 'Chain of evidence' are currently being produced by the Royal College of Pathologists. If a chain of evidence cannot be documented then courts may not accept findings from microbiological/virological investigations.

References

1   British Medical Association (2000) *Consent, Rights and Choices in Health Care for Children and Young People.* British Medical Association, London.
2   Department of Health (2001) *Reference Guide to Consent for Examination or Treatment.* Department of Health, London.
3   General Medical Council (2000) *Confidentiality: protecting and providing information.* General Medical Council, London.

4 Gillick v West Norfolk and Wisbech AHA [1986] AC 112, [1985] 3 WLR 830, [1985] 3 All ER 402, HL.

5 The NHS Trusts and Primary Care Trusts (Sexually Transmitted Diseases) Directions 2000 pursuant to Sections 17 and 126(3) of the National Health Service Act 1977(a).

6 *The Children Act 1989.* HMSO, London.

7 The European Convention on Human Rights 1950.

8 British Medical Association (2000) *The Impact of the Human Rights Act 1998 on Medical Decision-Making.* British Medical Association, London.

9 The Sexual Offences Reform Bill. Home Office; www.publications.parliament.uk

10 Thomas A, Forster G, Robinson A and Rogstad K (2002) National guidelines for the management of suspected sexually transmitted infections in children and young people. *Sex Transm Infect.* 78: 324–31.

11 The Victoria Climbie Enquiry; victoria-climbie-enquiry.org.uk

Appendix 4

Case summaries

To maintain confidentiality, the names of all patients have been changed.

Case A: 'Anne'

Age:	13 years.
Sex:	Female.
Culture:	White, British.
Education:	At school.
Home life:	Lives with her parents, who are both ill. Has a sister who lives nearby.
Appearance:	In tears, huddled in a chair and will not say what the problem is.
Setting:	Teenage GP practice clinic.
GP's sex:	Female.
GP's culture:	White.

Presenting problem

The mother called the nurse at the teenage clinic. Anne finds it difficult to attend school due to symptoms that appear to be psychosomatic. She is tearful.

Background information

Anne's father has MS and her mother has ME.

Subsequent consultations

This situation has not changed over the course of seven months and after the involvement of several health professionals, including the GP, practice nurse, psychiatrist, district nurse, health visitor and psychologist. However, although the GP feels that she is not communicating, the girl has by her actions managed to:

- draw attention to her unhappiness and be prescribed antidepressants which she is not averse to taking
- raise awareness of her situation at home
- acknowledge bullying at school, which is now resolved
- express concern about her periods and get the pill prescribed for her
- maintain regular contact with her GP, a concerned adult.

Case 1: 'Mary'

Age:	16 years.
Sex:	Female.
Culture:	White.
Education:	Not mentioned.
Home life:	Lives with her parents. Her mother suggested she should attend. No other mention of home life.
Appearance:	Seemed awkward and embarrassed.
Setting:	GP surgery.
GP's sex:	Female.
GP's culture:	White.

Presenting problem

Mary's mother suggested that she should visit the GP to get the pill for her acne.

Background

Mary said that someone had forced her to have sex once in the past. She was embarrassed to talk about sex. The GP felt that it was the mother's rather than the daughter's idea to come for the pill.

Subsequent consultations

A follow-up appointment was made for three months' time.

Case 2: 'Harold'

Age:	13 years.
Sex:	Male.
Culture:	Black, West Indian.
Education:	Suspended from school because he hit a teacher and acted inappropriately towards a girl pupil.
Home life:	Was brought up by his grandparents in the Caribbean, and was brought to England recently because of problems out there. His mother had remarried and had another child.
Appearance:	Not mentioned.
Setting:	GP surgery.
GP's sex:	Female.
GP's culture:	Black.

Presenting problem

The boy had been suspended from school. His mother wanted to know when he would be able to return, but the school was not answering her enquiries.

Background information

The boy had had some problem in the Caribbean, as well as problems settling at school.

Subsequent consultations

Not mentioned.

Case 3: 'Richard'

Age:	16 years.
Sex:	Male.
Culture:	White, British.
Education:	At college. Had done GCSEs, but on returning found studying difficult and had to reduce his workload.
Home life:	Lives at home with his mother and three sisters. The father is not at home and is not interested in discussing problems with him. One sister had a teenage pregnancy. The boy lives in a village, which makes it difficult for him to go out with his friends.
Appearance:	No strong impression.
Setting:	GP surgery.
GP's sex:	Female.
GP's culture:	White.

Presenting problem

Richard's mother took him to see the nurse at the teen clinic. He is suffering from insomnia and is aggressive and argumentative at home.

Background

The nurse at the teen clinic advised on conflict management and referred him to see the GP. He lives in an all-female environment. The mother has tried to involve the father or uncles but says that they are not interested.

Subsequent consultations

The GP suspected that the boy was depressed and prescribed an antidepressant with a sedative effect for his insomnia. The GP referred him to a child psychiatrist.

Case 4: 'Ann'

Age:	13 years.
Sex:	Female.
Culture:	White, British.
Education:	At school, but off school now because she is ill.
Home life:	Living with her parents.
Appearance:	No strong impression.
Setting:	GP surgery.
GP's sex:	Female.
GP's culture:	White.

Presenting problem

Her mother said that Ann would not go to school and was ill. She was not eating and her mother thought she might be anaemic. The GP tried to take a throat swab but she refused. The GP arranged a blood test.

Background information

Ann had been referred to child guidance four years previously after a problem subsequent to an accident at school.

Subsequent consultations

Ann returned for her test results, which were all clear. She discussed school and eating habits.

Case 5: 'Sally'

Age:	16 years.
Sex:	Female.
Culture:	White, British.
Education:	Not mentioned.
Home life:	Not mentioned.
Appearance:	Not mentioned.
Setting:	Child psychiatry unit.
Doctor's sex:	Female psychiatrist.
Doctor's culture:	White.

Presenting problem

Depression.

Background information

Not mentioned.

Subsequent consultations

The doctor was leaving the practice, and the girl did not want to transfer to another doctor.

Case 6: 'Gita'

This case was reported second-hand – not by the GP who saw the girl.

Age:	14 years.
Sex:	Female.
Culture:	Asian.
Education:	Not mentioned.
Home life:	Was being sexually abused at home.
Appearance:	Not mentioned.
Setting:	Teenage clinic.
Nurse's sex:	Female.
Nurse's culture:	White.

Presenting problem

Sexual abuse.

Background information

Not stated.

Subsequent consultations

Did not involve social services. Arranged follow-up appointments.

Case 7: 'Fatima'

Age:	16 years.
Sex:	Female.
Culture:	Asian, British.
Education:	At school, doing well.
Home life:	Initially lived with her mother and brother (who was head of the household because his father had died). She then moved in with another brother and his wife.
Appearance:	Not mentioned.
Setting:	Student health service.
GP's sex:	Female.
GP's culture:	Asian.

Presenting problem

The school counsellor thought Fatima was too thin and suggested that she had a check-up.

Background information

Fatima was seeing the counsellor because her family had discovered that she had a boyfriend and had 'gone mad about it'. She had moved out of her mother's home to her other married brother's house. He is schizophrenic, and a relapse led to problems with this new arrangement.

Subsequent consultations

Fatima returned to the GP to obtain her test results, and discussed problems at home. The GP felt that the situation was contained and that the school counsellor was acting as a 'safety-net'.

Case 8: 'Mary'

Age:	18 years.
Sex:	Female.
Culture:	White, British.
Education:	Had recently left school. Not academic, but able to help on her mother's vegetable stall.
Home life:	Living with her parents.
Appearance:	No strong impression.
Setting:	Long-term follow-up clinic.
GP's sex:	Male GP/consultant.
GP's culture:	White.

Presenting problem

Follow-up appointment after childhood cancer. Problem with finding a job.

Background information

Mary had been in hospital with cancer when aged 11 years, and had had a rough time. When she applied for school she was turned down on medical grounds. Her mother fought against this and she was eventually allowed to attend the school. She has now left school, but has failed to get jobs she has applied for, even though she felt that the interviews went well. She felt that this was due to prejudice relating to fear of cancer recurring again.

Subsequent consultations

The GP arranged a follow-up appointment and said that the hospital would write a letter to Mary's employers if they required a medical reference.

Case 9: 'Aisa'

Age:	18 years.
Sex:	Female.
Culture:	Asian.
Education:	In first year of university.
Home life:	Not mentioned.
Appearance:	No strong impression.
Setting:	Student health service.
GP's sex:	Female.
GP's culture:	Asian.

Presenting problem

Thrush.

Background information

Aisa had previously presented to the nurse with thrush, and presented to the GP with a recurrence.

Subsequent consultations

She had several contacts with the health services (two doctors and a nurse at the student health centre, an out-of-hours service doctor, and her home doctor). Her presenting problems were thrush and asthma. She did not disclose that she was pregnant (or worried about being so) until much later, when she was also found to have pelvic inflammatory disease. She then contacted the family planning clinic for a termination.

Case 10: 'Jyoti'

Age:	18 years.
Sex:	Female.
Culture:	Asian.
Education:	In her first year of college in London.
Home life:	Her family was still living in Leicester. She was living in university halls.
Appearance:	Well dressed, wearing trendy, noticeably tight trousers and quite a lot of make-up.
Setting:	Student health service.
GP's sex:	Female.
GP's culture:	White.

Presenting problem

Jyoti was seeking emergency contraception.

Background information

She had been investigated in the past because she believed herself to be very hairy (the GP did not think this was the case). She had been referred to an endocrinologist, who had found nothing but prescribed the pill.

Subsequent consultations

Jyoti came back presenting with thrush. It emerged that she felt caught between her Asian cultural background in Leicester and her life in London in a hall of residence. She had a non-Asian boyfriend and felt that she could not tell her parents about this relationship. She felt as if she was living two lives. When she went back home she had to be someone else. Her parents had found a husband for her and she was going to Toronto to meet him.

When she returned for a further prescription for the pill she was encouraged to have a smear. She was a little reluctant but agreed. On examination she flinched and the GP suspected that she had not actually had sex. When asked if she had had sex, she replied 'Oh yes', very unconvincingly.

At one further (final) consultation the GP was saying goodbye to her. As the girl was leaving, she said 'One more thing – I need emergency contraception.' The GP felt despairing and quite frustrated, especially as she was leaving the job and therefore would not have the chance to get to the bottom of the problem.

Appendix 5

Fraser Guidelines and codes of practice for health professionals

Fraser Guidelines

These are the Fraser Guidelines which were issued following a House of Lords' judgement in 1985. They relate to contraception but similar principles apply where other medical conditions are under consideration.

- The young person understands the doctor's advice.
- The doctor cannot persuade the young person to inform his or her parents to allow the doctor to inform the parents that he or she is seeking contraceptive advice.
- The young person is very likely to begin or continue having intercourse with or without contraceptive treatment.
- Unless he or she receives contraceptive advice or treatment, the young person's physical or mental health or both are likely to suffer.
- The young person's best interests require the doctor to give contraceptive advice, treatment or both without parental consent.

Codes of practice for health professionals

- Doctors, nurses and health professionals have a duty of confidentiality to patients of all ages, including under 16s.
- Only in exceptional circumstances may confidentiality be broken. Such a situation may arise if the health, safety or welfare of the patient, or others, would otherwise be at grave risk.
- The patient should be informed before confidentiality is broken, unless to do so would be dangerous to the patient or others.
- The steps which have been taken to obtain consent and the reasons for breaking confidentiality must be carefully documented.
- The health professionals must always be prepared to justify their decisions in accordance with the guidance from their professional bodies.

Further information can be found in:

- *Confidentiality and Young People: Improving teenagers' uptake of sexual and other health advice*, obtainable from the Royal College of General Practitioners.
- General Medical Council (2000) *Confidentiality: protecting and providing information*, pp. 17–18.

Index